AF887808

THE POSSIBILITIES ARE ENDLESS

by

Marsha Gabel Berman

TELEMACHUS PRESS

This book is a work of non-fiction. The events and characters are true, however, some or all of the names have been changed to protect personal identities. The events described are based on the recollection of the author and individual contributors as noted. Some persons may remember or interpret the persons, events and places described in this book differently.

Cover designed by Telemachus Press, LLC

Cover art:
Copyright © iStock-1224673700_traffic_analyzer_03cr.eps

Gamma Knife® is a registered trademark of Elekta Group

Published by Telemachus Press, LLC
7652 Sawmill Road
Suite 304
Dublin, Ohio 43016
http://www.telemachuspress.com

Visit the author website:
http://www.marshaberman.com

ISBN: 978-1-951744-49-6 (eBook)
ISBN: 978-1-951744-50-2 (Paperback)

Category: BIOGRAPHY & AUTOBIOGRAPHY / Medical

Version 2021.02.03

"It has been said that time heals all wounds.
I do not agree. The wounds remain.
In time, the mind protecting its sanity
Covers them with scar tissue and the pain lessens.
But it is never gone."

Rose Kennedy

ACKNOWLEDGEMENTS

I could go on forever but most of all I thank my family, our friends, my husband, Bobby and my son Dave and his family, and Jess and the boys. But most of all I with humble gratitude I want to acknowledge the doctors, hospitals, rehabs and all the medical personnel who cared for Brad. Their dedication was amazing and more grateful I could not be.

Of course, I want to thank Linda and Jay Spear who over and over edited and kept me focused as a new writer. Their skills are amazing and they put their faith in me.

Thank you, Linda and Jay.

DEDICATION

I dedicate this book to my son Brad, who endured so much pain and came out and healed and no mother could be more proud of their child. I knew from day one that he would fight to the end for the sake of his children and that is just what happened. His story is inspiring and brought healing to so many patients in his predicament.

TABLE OF CONTENTS

FOREWORD
Brad Berman

I am writing this exactly 2,039 days after I returned to the workforce following a grueling recovery from a catastrophic hemorrhage that left me in a coma for five weeks. That number matters to me because my odds of returning to a "normal" life where I would have a professional career and be able to care for myself and my family were basically zero.

I was always kind of a health nut. I watched what I ate and exercised a lot. I became obsessed with distance running because I knew I loved my ex-wife, Jessica, who is a runner when she told me that she wanted me to run a marathon with her. I found I was surprisingly good at it and enjoyed the physical discomfort that was a part of it, as well as the mental focus that it required.

In the autumn of 2013, five weeks after the stroke, I woke up in a hospital room and noticed that I had an awfully hard object inside of the right side of my abdomen and I could barely move the left side of my body. I soon learned that the hard object was the right side of my skull. A doctor decided to remove it in order to give my brain room to swell after the blood from a large hemorrhage began to create havoc. I felt a lot of pain on the left side of my body attributable to muscle tightness. I was disoriented and yearned for familiarity and comfort. The faces of my parents and my brother, Dave, brought me great comfort, but the face that made me feel safe was Jessica's.

I dealt with all kinds of rehabilitation with incredible therapists, but I couldn't grasp exactly what had happened to me. I always tried hard in the various therapies because I had tried hard at everything that I have done in my life. I tried hard out of pride and because my young kids, who were, and still are, my purpose. They watched me very closely.

I remember calling Jessica the "quarterback" of my recovery because she managed my rehab schedule, my medical team, my mental health, the equipment that I needed and much, much more, all while ensuring that our two young sons were safe and well cared for. She was Superwoman who did everything possible for me out of love. She ensured that while I was an in-patient for four months and while having several brain surgeries, I never had a problem with having our health insurer cover the expense. She also saw to all the expenses and that I was never alone in the hospital. She literally had a sign-up sheet to ensure I had company for every minute that I was awake. The two people who I trusted the most while I was struggling, were Jess and my brother, Dave. I trusted Jess because she was honest with me. She would admit that the situation was hard and bad while others tried to paint a rosier picture that I couldn't believe because I felt awful.

The press took notice of how Jess was raising hundreds of thousands of dollars to support my recovery and many news outlets wanted to interview me. The most enjoyable of all was meeting Irv Gitowsky, a meteorologist on a New York television station and radio, read about Brad and our family and made it his personal mission to follow his treatment and continuing labor to be well.

He came to my home with his wife and interviewed Jess, me, and the boys. Then he carried the story to his news broadcast and our struggle as well as our ongoing success caught the interest of his major television audience.

From then on Irv became a family member an often had dinner with us at Brad's house.

He even interviewed the boys in their bedroom. It was a sweet moment for his TV audience. They became such fast friends, that Brad and Jess were also invited to Irv's house for dinner as well.

Since he was also a marathon runner, he participated in the New York Marathon that year in our honor. It was a hopeful year and the beginning of a major fundraising campaign.

Jess ensured that I had amazing help when I got home from the hospital. She hired an aide named Joseph Brown, who became my caregiver and remains like a brother to me today.

Recovering from a brain injury is 100 percent consuming. I once told my incredible neurosurgeon that it feels like going through life with somebody playing defense against you. However, you learn how to navigate it with time. You just have to run over obstacles.

I am lucky. I recovered from something that kills most people who experience it. Although I survived, my marriage didn't. Jess and I split up in 2019. Although that part was sad, we grew apart and were able to separate while remaining close friends and very cooperative co-parents to our sons. Our relationship is forever bound by respect, admiration, and a commitment to put our sons first.

I have a new life and am incredibly blessed. My sons are healthy, smart, empathic, and athletic. My friends and family stood by my side without exception. My parents are perfect and teach me so much to this day. My girlfriend, Diana, is an absolutely incredible, beautiful human being. She has faced serious health challenges of her own and we are strong together. Her kindness and warm heart shifted me from recovering, back to living. I am in a unique position to advise dozens of people who have suffered injuries similar to mine. Doing that has become especially important to me.

My lessons learned from my experience are to never quit on yourself, be humble and kind. You never know what somebody is going through in their life.

But, enough about me. The rest of the story will be told by the woman who stood by me from day one, protected me, spent countless hours at the hospital and in rehab. She worried about me and loved me no matter what. We don't get to choose our mothers, but I got the best one. As a parent myself, I can't imagine what my mom felt as she watched me suffer. I admire her strength and determination to tell her story and I love her with all of my heart.

Lucky me.

THE POSSIBILITIES ARE ENDLESS

CHAPTER ONE

I HUGGED MY new baby and very slowly rocked him back and forth. While I held him, I would whisper the old adage:

I will love you forever
I will like you for always
As long as I am living
My baby you will be.

The baby grew tall and strong and by the time he was two, he ran all around the house and pulled books off of shelves to be read to him. Every night, when he was asleep, I would quietly open the door to his room and begin to whisper his favorite lullaby again.

And so it went throughout his childhood. He grew to be an exemplary person and I was as proud as a parent could be. Things could not have been better for him. But on August 4, 2013, my first-born, Brad, reached the threshold of death at age 37. My family and I were hit with what only could be described as a tidal wave of emotional and soul wrenching pain. My son was dying and there was nothing any of us, at least in the initial moments, could do to alter the outcome.

CHAPTER TWO

THERE ARE TIMES when life takes us on unexpected trips where we have little or no control over destiny. This was one of those moments. Over the course of minutes, hours, days, weeks, months, and years, we were left in the sometimes kind and sometimes cruel hands of fate. The future took us on a roller coaster ride beyond our control.

This is a story of luck, kindness, hopelessness, faith, and love. If I tried to explain why each step along the way occurred, I am not sure that would be possible.

We have no choice but to reset our lives when triggered. Being able to quickly change course becomes your immediate priority. It is truly a reflection of ourselves. You must clear your mind every day, you cannot ignore your feelings, or they will control your emotions beyond your ability to restrain the hardship.

Families need to talk and set their intentions for the day and the weeks ahead as much as possible because it is your strength that is needed to make your plan work.

Do not be defensive and do not make it about yourself.

Being in the fight and flight mode for too long, wreaks havoc on our bodies.

Try to help compassionately and create solutions instead of complaining and finger pointing.

We all have a choice, and it all starts with us and our willingness to take action, today.

The following account is what happened to my family and friends who watched, waited, and finally moved forward. Beginnings are scary; endings are often sad. Fortunately, it is the middle that counts the most. I learned on August 4th of 2013 to give hope a chance for an ending to a terrifying experience. At age 37, my older son was struck down by a catastrophic brain hemorrhage. But what could have caused it?

We soon found out.

CHAPTER THREE

A STROKE WAS the last thing Jessica Berman suspected when her husband frantically called her while she was exercising at a local fitness center, telling her to come home. Fortunately, she had her cell phone in her hand.

To her, Brad Berman was the embodiment of great health. He ate a balanced diet, exercised regularly, and was a marathon runner. He was successful, working as a Vice president and Tax Director at GE Asset Management. Brad was as strong and vital as a young man could possibly be.

That fateful morning, he dressed for a run, in preparation for the upcoming New York City Marathon. As he reached the kitchen, Brad's headache began to worsen, and he knew something was terribly wrong. As he spoke to his wife on the phone, she was shocked by his garbled speech, and knew there was a disaster in progress. Jessica sped home to find Brad lying on the kitchen floor. Brad was having a stroke, a medical emergency that claims almost 130,000 lives each year in the United States.

"Brad is the healthiest person I know. I could have never imagined that he was having a stroke," Jessica, his wife of nine years, told the local news stations and newspapers when the companies heard about Brad's plight.

Jessica immediately called the local ambulance and Brad, now unconscious, was transported to the small local hospital's Emergency Room. We followed behind in a cab. No one knew what to expect when Brad was wheeled into the hospital and switched from the gurney onto a hospital bed.

There lay what was obviously once a strong and vital man with lean musculature and a tanned body.

It was obvious from the onset that Brad needed more extensive support than he could receive there, and he was immediately transferred to Westchester Medical Center in Valhalla, NY.

The cause of an AVM is unclear. Arteries are responsible for taking oxygen rich blood from the heart to the brain. Veins carry the oxygen-depleted blood back to the lungs and heart. When an AVM disrupts this critical process, the surrounding tissues may not get enough oxygen, and the affected arteries and veins can weaken and rupture.

Early on, AVMs, although not inherited, are not visible at birth because they would be too small to see. It's unfortunate that they are often discovered in tragic ways.

Dr. Avinash Mohan, Chief of Neurosurgery at Westchester Medical Center, was immediately called. He reviewed all the information and performed a physical exam. Then he listened for a sound called bruit. Bruit is a whooshing sound caused by very rapid blood flow through the arteries and veins of an AVM. It sounds like water rushing through a narrow pipe.

The tests used to help diagnose Brad's AVM included a cerebral angiography. Also called an arteriography. This test uses a special dye called a contrast agent injected into an artery. The dye highlights the structure of blood vessels to better show them on X-rays. A computerized tomography (CT) otherwise known as Cat Scans use X-rays to create images of the head, brain or spinal cord and can help to show bleeding.

Magnetic resonance imaging (MRI) which uses powerful magnets and radio waves to show detailed images of the tissues, can pick up on small changes in these tissues. Magnetic resonance angiography (MRA) captures the pattern and the speed and distance of blood flow through the vascular abnormalities was used as was a Transcranial Doppler ultrasound. This type of ultrasound uses high-frequency sound waves to create an image of the blood flow to help diagnose large and medium AVMs, as well as bleeding.

It was clear to Dr. Mohan that surgery needed to be immediately performed. He carefully explained the diagnosis to Jessica, Bobby, and me, obtained our consent, and performed a craniotomy, removing a portion of Brad's skull then carefully storing it in his abdomen. This procedure is routine for cases such as this and it relieves the immense pressure caused by the swelling in Brad's brain. After surgery, Brad was stable, and was placed in a medically induced coma that he would remain in for over a month. It was decided that he would ultimately be transferred to a rehabilitation facility.

At this point, we felt we had to update close friends and family about what was going on. Other family members and friends were devastated as well. My sister-in-law, Maddy, my sister-in-law, was on vacation with her husband, Richie, when I first spoke to her.

They were in Plymouth, Massachusetts visiting friends. Of course, they were in shock, as they left to go home feeling tense and overwhelmed.

Shortly thereafter, Jeanette Berman, my mother-in-law, learned of the situation and was shattered when she reflected on Brad's condition.

"When I saw Brad, it almost tore me apart. He is Bobby's first child. It was so difficult for me to see him in that condition. His Poppa Sid, who was my husband, would have been literally crushed to witness what happened to Brad. We both adored him."

Once Dr. Mohan felt Brad was sufficiently stable following the surgery, he was eager to get intensive rehabilitation efforts started. It was decided that Brad would be transferred to Helen Hayes Rehabilitation Center, in Haverstraw, NY when he was sufficiently healed from the attack and surgery. No one knew how long that would take, but our hopes were high as we took our cues from the positive nature of the people who cared for him.

While still in the ICU at Westchester Medical Center, five weeks later, Brad started to awaken. It was a gradual occurrence. He opened his eyes, would sometimes respond to verbal commands to give a thumbs up, to snap his fingers, or even give a high five and then close his eyes and rest for quite a while.

During this five-week-long period, we learned more about an AVM than one can handle and that was quite frightening. We heard all the possibilities that could come of this absolute disaster. No parent can stand to see their child suffer and we suffered all the more when we learned that we were far from recovery.

During that initial month, it was like a crash course in a topic you would hope you never have to learn. It made us feel like we had little control over Brad's health or even our own. We learned that AVMs are not genetically caused but could be recognized at birth. They could lay dormant for someone's entire life. It could also be discovered before rupturing and treated with successful results. Or it could never be discovered until it had already resulted in a significant brain bleed which can be deadly.

We dealt with grief with our hearts wide open. Strength, hope, and determination were words we lived by. I knew I would walk through fire dedicating myself to ensure that my son got when he needed to be well again.

Every day, after Bobby went to work, I arrived at the hospital by 10 am. I would spend at least one hour praying for Brad's recovery. There were three chapels for the three major religions, and I went to each one, knowing that God was listening to me wherever I was.

I lit candles and prayed as hard as a mother could for the recovery of her child at any age he was. It affected my life and my soul in the deepest way possible. It takes patience and I forged ahead. I was obsessed with his chance of recovery. After praying, I would walk straight to his room. After a week or less of performing this routine, I could have gotten there blindfolded.

Because of the shift work, Jennifer, his primary nurse, was available to him for only three days a week, but we adapted to every day as different professionals took exceptional care of him. Nowadays, when people refer to those on "the front line," I am more aware of their importance than ever before.

As time went by, Brad's ability to speak changed. My routine early in the morning remained the same in the three chapels available in the hospital, but I always arrived in his room on time to attend his therapy sessions, and never held back in seeing that he got all the services and attention he needed.

The fear, however, never left me, and I felt utter panic throughout our time in the hospital. Still, I could not pull myself away. The depth of my feelings became apparent to those who took care of him and some of his caretakers were very empathic. I was not, however, afraid to speak up about his care about those who were not. I realized that my son could not be left alone, so when no other family member was there, I would be.

Jessica coordinated the schedule and made it a priority that Brad was never without a friend or family member by his side.

As a result, I became a new person—one I never knew or expected to come forward. I have always been quiet, but when my child was threatened, my ferocity came through and I battled through thick and thin. It takes patience and strength to forge ahead. I wanted that child's AVM to be mine and as long as I live, I will always feel that way. I felt I had lived a good life, and my child needed to continue his life throughout his growth in manhood.

In my world, it was not natural for Brad to be sick. His illness was not something I could bear to suffer, yet I hoped every day that the course would change.

I knew every day, with his own energy, Brad would resume his pre-stroke abilities and get back to himself for the sake of himself and his family. He received exemplary treatment for the most part, as loving care is a spectacular resource of WCMC and Helen Hayes and other excellent hospitals. but I could not pull myself away, for fear that something might go awry.

CHAPTER FOUR

EARLY ON, BRAD was still at a high risk of more intensive bleeding. Recovering from the AVM rupture was only a piece of the puzzle. As long as the AVM remained in Brad's brain, he was at risk of recurring bleeds. There were various options explained to us, including major brain surgery to remove the AVM. However, typically this treatment is used when it is still small and located in an area where surgeons can remove it with little risk of causing significant damage to the brain tissues.

Endovascular embolization is initially used routinely for this type of situation. It is a procedure in which the surgeon threads a catheter through the arteries to the AVM. Next, a substance is injected to create an artificial blood clot in the middle of the AVM to temporarily reduce the blood flow. Once this has been done to stabilize the blood vessels, the surgery to remove the AVM then follows.

In other situations, stereotactic radiosurgery is used. This procedure is usually performed on small AVMs that have not ruptured but is utilized in other situations as well. The machine called the Gamma Knife® uses intense, highly focused beams of radiation to damage the blood vessels and stop the blood supply to the AVM.

While we were so impressed with the team that cared for Brad and had put our trust in Dr. Mohan and his team at Westchester Medical Center, we knew we had to get input from other brilliant minds around the country on the best option for our son. It was the major reason why Brad regained his ability to walk and heal.

Jessica and Dave put all of their efforts into getting to the best and brightest neurosurgeons in the country to express an opinion. Their quest was satisfying when they found the best surgeon in our country to use the Gamma Knife that made all the difference.

CHAPTER FIVE

THROUGHOUT THIS NEXT challenging and stressful phase, I was reminded of the Coldplay lyrics to *Fix You*, which describe someone in deep struggles being guided to a safe place, filled with hope when none seemed to exist before and then comforted. At times it seemed like the lyrics were describing our situation perfectly and gave us comfort.

I quickly learned that the current treatment for AVM depends on where the abnormality is found, the symptoms that you have, and your overall health. Sometimes, an AVM may be monitored with regular imaging tests to watch for changes or problems.

Although medications can help manage symptoms such as seizures, headaches, and back pain, yet leave him helpless, Dr. Mohan was determined to improve Brad's chances of returning to health.

Our biggest fear was that Brad was at high risk of more intensive bleeding. Recovering from the AVM rupture was only one piece of the puzzle. As long as the AVM remained in Brad's brain, he was at risk of recurring bleeds. There were various options explained to us, including major brain surgery to remove the AVM. However, this treatment is typically used when the AVM is still small and located in an area where surgeons can remove it with little risk of causing significant damage to the brain tissues.

In other situations, stereotactic radiosurgery is used. This procedure is usually performed on small AVMs that have not ruptured but is utilized in other situations as well. A machine called the Gamma Knife uses intense, highly focused beams of radiation to damage the blood vessels and stop the blood supply to the AVM.

While we were so impressed and had put our trust in Dr. Mohan and his team at Westchester Medical Center, we knew we had to get input from other brilliant minds across the country as to the best option for Brad.

Jessica put all of her efforts into finding the best specialists and speaking to them, wherever they were. David, Brad's younger brother, remembers what he refers to as the most stressful day of his life when he accompanied Jessica on this quest.

It was in the Fall of 2013 when Jessica arranged appointments at Columbia and NYU on the very same day. David met with the prestigious Columbia team of neurosurgeons who told him that surgery was the only answer. He was also told that if we relied on the radiation with the Gamma Knife, that Brad would likely rebleed and possibly die.

David then raced to find a cab to take him down to NYU where he met with Jessica. There, they were told that while surgery was certainly an option, the risks were high. Brad could end up paralyzed and unable to walk again. Or he could bleed out on the table. Their proposal was for radiation with the Gamma Knife: Jessica and Dave were faced with two starkly different and competing proposals from two renowned institutions within blocks of each other, in a matter of hours.

I jumped in a cab and went from Westchester Medical Center all the way down to NYU to meet Jessica and Dave and the chief of the neurosurgical team. There we were told that the surgery would paralyze or kill him. Gamma, however, was their choice and Dr. Kondziolka who was chief of stereotactic and functional neurosurgery and director of the Center for Brain Function and Behavior at the University of Pittsburgh before joining the staff of NYU's neurosurgical staff was chosen because he made all the difference in the treatment of Brad's condition.

When we returned to Westchester that day, we met with Brad's surgical team at the Medical Center and they said that they could not do either.

"Take him home," the team concurred, "and do nothing. Let him live his life and hope the AVM does not re-bleed."

Jess, Dave, Bobby, and I put our heads together and all agreed that this was not our choice and the Gamma Knife surgery made the most sense of it all before it became too late.

Dr. Howard Riina was the lead neurosurgeon and his colleague, Dr. Kondziolka was the pre-eminent expert in the field of Gamma Knife surgery. In December 2013, Brad had his first Gamma Knife treatment.

Gamma Knife radiosurgery is one of the most advanced and non-invasive options for brain-related conditions like, malignant and benign brain tumors, arteriovenous malformations, tremor due to essential tremor or Parkinson's disease and trigeminal neuralgia.

Since it is an outpatient procedure, Gamma Knife patients are able to return home the same day, with a reduced recovery time versus that of conventional brain surgery. Brad was lucky to have Dr. Douglas Kondzoilka at Langone who is currently the world's leading expert in Gamma Knife radiation.

He told us that he joined NYU Langone's neurosurgery faculty as a professor and vice chair of clinical research in 2012.

"In addition to performing research and training neurosurgeons, I treat patients who have neurological conditions, such as metastatic brain tumors, acoustic neuroma (also known as vestibular schwannoma), meningioma, primary brain tumors, brain vascular malformations, movement and behavioral disorders, and trigeminal neuralgia. I am also director of the Center for Advanced Radiosurgery, where we treat patients with Gamma Knife.

"Prior to coming to NYU Langone, I also served as the vice chair for education and the neuroscience task force leader for the McGowan Institute for Regenerative Medicine. I worked with the National Hockey League's Pittsburgh Penguins from 2002 to 2012 as their neurosurgeon. As the principal investigator of the first two clinical trials for patients who had experienced strokes and was the co-principal investigator of a third clinical trial on bone marrow–derived neuroprogenitor cell implantation for stroke.

"I have also completed two clinical trials in neurostimulation research for major depression and have launched the first global registry platform for neurosurgery, which focuses on a range of conditions managed with radiosurgery. My current laboratory and clinical research into stereotactic radiosurgery spans many conditions, including benign and malignant tumors, vascular malformations, and functional disorders.

"In addition to conducting research and treating patients, I have published 480 journal articles and 250 book chapters, and I've edited eight books. I have also served as the co-chair of the editorial board of the *Journal of Neurosurgery* and am now the associate editor of the journal, and presently a director of the American Board of Neurological Surgery."

One can understand why we chose him to perform the Gamma Knife procedure. The treatments that Dr. Kondziolka performs are a well-established and widely recognized options in use around the world and they are approved for use by the U.S. Food and Drug Administration. How lucky we were to have found him.

At Langone, more than 30,000 patients undergo Gamma Knife treatment each year. While it is most commonly used to treat brain metastases, it may also be used as a therapy for primary and benign brain tumors, trigeminal neuralgia, arteriovenous malformations, and certain movement disorders.

For Gamma Knife radiosurgery, a single one- to two-hour treatment is typically required, in which 192 beams of gamma rays are focused on multiple points throughout the target with the aim of matching the delivered radiation to the shape of the tumor.

Thus, the gamma radiation is concentrated in the area, minimizing radiation to tissue lying in the entry or exit pathways. Because of this precise focusing ability, aggressive, high-dose gamma radiation can be delivered to stabilize, shrink, or destroy some lesions—even those deep in the cerebral hemispheres or brain stem.

For many patients, this computer-guided therapy can deliver targeted radiation to reduce tumors and lesions deep within the brain with pinpoint accuracy that cannot be matched by traditional surgery.

What is more, this outpatient procedure is nearly painless and requires no incisions. Just think about the historical record of the treatment for brain disfunction and then imagine brain surgery without pain!

After each Gamma Knife treatment, Brad required an angiogram to spot any deficiencies. This part was more difficult than the Gamma process. Brad was required to lay still with extraordinarily little movement for six hours to ensure recuperation followed by an angiogram and an MRI to determine the success of the procedure.

Since the usual time for the Gamma Knife to work is five years, but miraculously, Brad's AVM had wholly disappeared by July 2015. This is the lucky part of his story. To hear that it had been totally obliterated was wonderful, but it was still so hard on Brad who looked at me and nodded when I hugged him with joy.

But Brad looked at me with sadness—this was something unusual for him.

"It's gone but it already did its damage," he said.

I did not understand the depth of his remark. That came years later.

CHAPTER SIX

BRAD TOLD ME shortly after his Gamma Knife surgery that looking back eight years ago, on August 4, 2013, it is impossible to imagine what actually happened to him. At that time, he said, he was successful with his career, his family life was great, and I had become an accomplished marathon runner. In my estimation, it was a perfect life.

According to Brad: Early that morning, he woke up with a massive headache and decided to go downstairs to get some water because he was thirsty as well. Jessica, his wife, had already left for the gym and their two sons were still asleep. He planned to give the boy's breakfast while their mother was out, but the headache increased to seismic proportions. It was the worst pain he had ever endured in his entire life.

Suddenly, he felt himself falling and yet he managed not to strike his head on the kitchen floor. At virtually the very same time, I called Jessica who, by chance, had her cell phone in her hand and heard his cry for help.

It took less than five minutes for her to run in the door and find his flailing body trying to get up. He awkwardly told her he was in trouble and she instantly called for an ambulance and EMTs.

She knelt down beside him and without thinking any further, he told her where to find his insurance card. But before she went to retrieve it, she called our parents and put them on alert.

The EMTs were swift and efficient and they hoisted him onto a gurney and into the ambulance. The plan was to ultimately get me to the closest hospital, but Westchester Medical Hospital, which is an exemplary establishment and close to where we lived, was where we ended up.

Jessica rode with us and kept both sets of our parents informed. She also asked her best friend Melissa, to take their boys back to her house. Melissa assured Jessica that she would take them to their favorite diner for breakfast and would care for them for whatever time thereafter she was needed. That is what a good friend does, and I will always appreciate her love for Jess and the rest of us. I understand that once the boys were finished with their meal, Brad's dad picked them up, and took the children to their home.

During this time, Brad heard bits and pieces of these phone conversations, but je suffered brutal seizures and from that point on, he heard nothing more for over a month.

By then, Brad had entered a coma.

Natalie Dawn, the EMT nurse who we found out later was Brad's exact age, yelled out to Jessica as Natalie pumped my heart, "I won't let him die," she whispered, and she did not. She worked on Brad for close to a half hour to keep his heart pumping and she only stopped when they reached the hospital and the emergency staff rushed out to take over.

Brad knew nothing of this and frankly, neither did I. I also recalled nothing of walking into the hospital. In fact, I was in such a state of shock that my first memories of the incident were when I was allowed to enter to Westchester Medical Center with my husband, Bobby, my son Dave and his wife, Vanessa to see Brad.

From early on, Brad was always surrounded by those who cared. To this day, he tells me he wished he could have seen this army of support encircling me before he began treatment.

Within the first month, Brad was given all the tests necessary to ensure what the medical staff believed had happened to him and what further treatment should begin.

Our friend and in-law, an interventional radiologist, Ron Aboody, joined us at the hospital and read my x-rays, charts and labs and agreed with the chief of neurosurgery at Westchester Medical, that Brad needed immediate brain surgery.

Dave was told that Dr. Avi Mohan had a brother the very same age as me and another brother the same age as him. He viewed Brad with a kind of protective custody. During the lengthy surgery, he removed the left section of my skull—which had been devastated by the stroke. Then he nested it in the soft tissue of my abdomen to keep in in viable condition to be placed back in my brain soon after.

Dr. Mohan is a Neurosurgery Specialist with offices in Hawthorne, NY, and has over 19 years of experience in the medical field. He has more experience with Cranial Neurosurgery than many other specialists in our region.

He graduated from Case Western Reserve University School of Medicine medical school in 2001. He is affiliated with medical facilities Vassar Brothers Medical Center and Westchester Medical Center.

Dr. Mohan is also a pediatric neurosurgeon. He specializes in treating and caring for children with complex neurological conditions and injuries. Dr. Mohan is extensively involved with teaching within the Neurological Surgery and Pediatrics Department of New York Medical College.

That side of the brain controls the right side of my body was the one that was affected. If all went well, Brad's brain would be working as before. But before my family could get their hopes up, Brad did not awake from the coma for five weeks following the surgery. This factor is not unusual, yet it makes the likelihood of a full remission from the incident quite unlikely.

With little else for then to do for me other than pray and visit me in the hospital as well as the Burke Rehabilitation Center later in his recovery. We were encouraged by more and more good news and the tremendous strides he made toward recovery with every ounce of grit and determination anyone could have. They already knew that he would fight for his life and find his way through the fight for his life.

CHAPTER SEVEN

THERE WERE TIMES during the month that Brad was in a medically induced coma when he looked lifeless, and we worried all the more. However, very gradually, we began to see him awaken. I walked the halls of Westchester Medical Center when I wasn't caring for my son and kept a watchful eye on the physical and occupational therapists as they helped him move his body in the bed and dangle his feet to the floor.

My brother and Brad's uncle, Larry Gabel, was overwhelmed when he learned the news.

"We received an email from my brother-in-law, that our nephew, Brad had been rushed to the hospital and was in a coma. How could a 37-year-old man be in that condition? But my first thought was that someone hacked his email account. We learned soon enough that it wasn't as easy as a mistake that Google could fix."

Larry came to see his nephew, and my brother was particularly taken aback as his first sight of his listless, shriveled, and bedridden body.

"I do not normally have a strong stomach for hospital visits in the first place," said Larry, "but the actual sight of him attached to life support and countless wires and tubes with one side of his head looking as though it had collapsed into itself was unspeakably shocking. I felt like I had actually been punched in the gut.

"I remember Marsha saying that I should leave the room if I could not handle it, but I felt as though my feet were glued to the floor.

"I was only 19 when Brad was born, and I babysat for him a few times when he was incredibly young—marveling at how Marsha and Bobby could have trusted me—a young guy who knew nothing about babies. I remember worrying about how to take care of this little guy. But as time went on, I loved him all the more. When he was a toddler, I introduced him to my wife to be and he became the ring bearer at our wedding.

"As he grew, I used to play-wrestle with this sturdy kid, as my wife and I watched him grow up and have kids of his own. He surely found his stride in life and was the picture of health. How could this be happening to him?"

With little else for us to do for him other than pray and visit him in the hospital as well as the Burke Rehabilitation Center later in his recovery. We. as a family, were encouraged by more and more good news and the tremendous strides he made toward recovery with every ounce of grit and determination one could have. We already knew that Brad would fight for his life and find his way through the terrible ordeal.

Adam Berman, Richie's son, totally agreed. "I have very vivid memories of the day Brad had his stroke as well as some of the visits we made to both Westchester Medical Center and Burke Rehab. I remember getting a call on a Sunday morning in early August saying that Brad was in the hospital with a brain injury. Not many details available at that time so the concern was great. My mind was consumed with the situation as we waited for more info and hopefully some good news. By the end of the day we learned he had suffered a major stroke and was in a coma—not the good news we were hoping to hear.

"The first visit I made to the hospital was just a few days later. I felt compelled to be there by his side to provide encouragement and support to him as well as his family. It was devastating to see this bright, funny, caring person in this state, but he was alive and that brought me and all of us some hope.

"I made a few other visits to the hospital with my wife and children during this time. Each visit was a bit sobering to see him that way and to see the concern on the faces of his family, but he was getting great care and we all knew he would not give up.

"Eventually his condition began to improve, and he came out of the coma. What a relief for all! Now the hard part began. What would come next? What does recovery truly mean for him? What will be his quality of life? How will Jess and his boys deal with the situation? I think Brad surprised us all as his recovery has been nothing short of remarkable. Each subsequent visit or phone call was more encouraging than the last. Brad's talking, remembering things, learning to walk again, and best of all joking around again.

"One afternoon, we brought lunch to Burke rehab and I remember him being fixated on a football player that had been in the news—Richie Incognito—and I was amazed that he could even pronounce that name after all he had been through. Good sign and a large wave of relief penetrated the room.

"Over the past few years we continued to see huge signs of recovery. Back to work, driving, cursing the moves the New York Giants make, and being a devoted father.

"It has been a long road for Brad but one he always seems to handle with grace and courage. Thanks for coming back to us Brad."

Carrie Poole, Adam's sister, and Richie's daughter agreed.

"When I saw Brad in the ICU in an induced coma, I just wondered how he would feel when he could comprehend what had happened to him. Would he be angry, scared, confused, cheated? I'm sure he went through all different kinds of emotions during his recovery, but all I have seen is a strong, tenacious, loving person who would do anything for his two boys."

CHAPTER EIGHT

BRAD: FORTUNATELY, I awoke from the coma before I arrived at the Helen Hayes Rehabilitation center in Haverstraw, NY, where three rehab nurses, plus several doctors began to help bring me back to my senses again. It was there that I learned that I had suffered a grade five AVM which had given me a slim to no chance at all to live. When I was able to stand again after months of treatment, I weighed less than 120 pounds. For a man who is almost six feet tall, I must have looked like a skin-covered skeleton!

The first thing the doctors did was administer a Glasgow Coma Scale which is a neurological testing device that aims to give a reliable and objective way of recording the state of a person's consciousness for initial as well as subsequent brain function assessment. A person's awareness is assessed against the criteria of the scale, and the resulting points give a person's score between three (indicating deep unconsciousness) and either fourteen (original scale) or fifteen (the more widely used and more modified scale).

The GCS scale is now used by emergency medical services and nurses as being applicable to all acute medical and trauma patients. In hospitals, it is also used in monitoring patients intensive care units. And believe it or not, despite all my body had been through, I passed the test!

With the fact that I was on my feet again and gaining ground every day with physical, occupational, and other types of therapy. Soon, I was ready to have the section of my skull, still resting in my abdomen, removed, and put back in place. That is when it became time for me to go to Langone New

York University Hospital for a cranioplasty where my strength and potential to live would be tested.

Dr. Howard Riina chose to pursue a career in neurosurgery because he wanted to help people and was drawn to patient care and treatment innovation. He performed the cranioplasty by putting the piece of skull back to my brain.

"It seems a lot is said these days about resilience and grit," said Dr. Riina. "A whole academic science has grown up around the factors and traits that allow a person to succeed. But this toughness is often measured in scholastic or career achievement and pales in comparison to what we observe in individuals who must triumph over a life altering calamity."

"Faced with a catastrophic series of events including an AVM hemorrhage, coma and hemiparesis (partial paralysis), Brad demonstrated a mental toughness and drive that is not seen in most people. Consider what it takes to teach yourself from day one of recovery to be independent, to feed yourself, dress yourself and walk. Then consider what it takes to return to work in your chosen career. You might—and I say might—have some idea of the grit that Brad Berman has demonstrated," acknowledged Dr. Riina as he shook his head in amazement.

All of the replacement surgery was done at NYU Langone Medical Center which is an academic medical hub located in New York City, New York, United States. It is also affiliated with New York University.

The Medical Center comprises the NYU School of Medicine and several hospitals: Tisch Hospital, the Rusk Institute of Rehabilitation Medicine, the Hospital for Joint Diseases, NYU Langone Hospital—Brooklyn, NYU Winthrop Hospital, and most recently, Hassenfeld Children's Hospital. NYU Langone Medical Center also operates over thirty ambulatory facilities in Manhattan, Brooklyn, Queens, and Long Island!

In early 2016, NYU Langone had approximately 25,000 employees, and over 8,000 more employees were gained after the acquisition of Long Island's center. The main campus of NYU Langone Medical Center overlooks the East River.

It was placed on the Honor Roll of *U.S. News & World Report* "Best Hospitals" in the nation for 2012-2015 and was named the #12 Hospital in the nation on the 2015-2016 "Best Hospitals" Honor Roll.

In the 2016-2017 rankings, NYU Langone claimed the number 10 spot, overtaking Barnes-Jewish Hospital of Washington University in St. Louis. In 2019, the hospital was once again moved up the list to the #9 hospital in the U.S.

At NYU Langone, Dr. Riina, who specializes in surgical and endovascular treatment for people who have cerebrovascular disorders of the brain and spinal cord, was first to examine Brad after he awoke from the surgery.

Cerebrovascular conditions are those that affect the blood vessels and blood flow to the brain and spinal cord. This includes patients with stroke, ruptured and unruptured brain aneurysms, and carotid disease, as well as vascular malformations and that was me.

Dr. Riina collaborates with neurologists, neuro-radiologists, and neuro-rehabilitation specialists to treat people who have had strokes and other complex neurovascular conditions at NYU Langone's Center for Stroke and Neurovascular Diseases. His approach is cooperative, and he treats patients by providing expertise in all aspects of their care. By working together, they are able to improve patient outcomes and treat lesions that are often thought to be untreatable or thought to be associated with a poor prognosis like mine. "We also focus on patient-centered care, with the goal of embracing our patients and their families by keeping them involved and informed during every aspect of their treatment."

I believe that Dr. Riina's emotional response to Brad was equally as important as his technological brilliance. Nothing was more of the truth. He learned that as time went on and hard work ensued for him, research for doctors is the key to better medicine.

CHAPTER NINE

SUMMER 2004. THAT year was sublime. The children were grown and developing their own skill sets to manage the rest of their lives. Bobby and I were looking at our home in Yorktown Heights with the notion that it had become too large for our needs. We lived in that house until both of our sons moved on.

This is the case with many people we knew who were our age and living in empty nests. Brad and his girlfriend Jessica were living together, and Dave was living with his girlfriend, Vanessa. Engagements and weddings followed.

Eventually, Brad and Jess' first child, Noah, was born in 2008. He was so sweet and cuddly. Imagine the joy a first grandchild brings to you? The new family was living and working in New York City and I stayed a while at their apartment to help them until they found support service for two working parents of a baby.

That is when Pinky came into their lives in as a Nanny. What joy she brought to the young family with Noah. Pinky loved them all and everyone was overjoyed with the happiness the whole family experienced.

"From the best of my knowledge when you meet good people you don't lose them," Pinky said. "They bring out the best in others. I helped Brad and Jess when they lived in the city, but when they moved to Larchmont, I had to leave my employment with them because I lived too far away in Queens and I don't drive. I left when Noah was two and I miss them all to this day. They are humble, joyful, compassionate, and loving people. A person with a good heart like Brad's keep you beautiful inside forever. We remain in touch and my heart always misses him when I leave to go to another job."

Bobby and I were the lucky ones as we worked at in careers that we both loved—I, as the manager of a medical office and Bobby in finance. We moved to our beautiful condo over ten years ago and were living a serene life. We also traveled the world with and without the children. That beautiful existence continued through August 2013 until Brad fell ill and that is when our life's work became the urgency to help our son survive.

From that moment on, I put our lives on hold and went into motion for Brad's recovery. I remember one day in the beginning of the siege, I decided to take a day off for some rest. It was that one day when he fell during physical therapy. From that point on, I never missed a day with him, and my own routine became to bathe and dress, have a quick breakfast, stop at a local café to pick up lunch and go to whatever hospital or rehab Brad was in and stay there until at least four in the afternoon. I hated to leave him there, fearing something else would happen while I was away.

Brad was at Westchester Medical Center for over five weeks, The Helen Hayes Rehab Center for six weeks, another week in NYU Langone to have more surgery and six more weeks in Burke Rehabilitation Center.

During this period of time, Brad went from a coma and virtual lifelessness to an awakened state with eyes wide open and curiosity beaming from them. He would listen to music he loved, eat well, dangle his legs, and engage in some arduous physical and occupational therapy until he was standing and able to walk with a cane.

Life through us a bunch of curves and with them all came a quirky semblance of order.

All in all, Brad was hospitalized for four full months, until December fourth, when he was able to come home. Outpatient rehab followed at Burke until the Christmas break and then it continued into the new year.

That is when Valrie came into the lives of Jess, Brad, and Noah when Noah was almost two. Andrew was born in 2010 and Joseph, physical therapist came into the household in December 2013 after Brad was released from in-patient Burke.

Valrie was the children's nanny of their two young sons, ages four and a half and two and a half and worked alongside Joseph when Andrew was born two years later. She and Joseph made a dream team for the beleaguered family. Said Valrie: "I was devastated to hear that Brad fell ill, but I had the chance to go visit him in the hospital and I was moved to tears and felt so dismayed when I saw him hooked up to the medical machines. At first, I thought he was dead, and I remember praying to God to work a miracle on him since the boys needed him in their lives. Clearly, God helped the doctors do a great job with Brad and he survived."

But we needed more help. Burke nurses recommended a man by the name of Joseph Brown to live in their new home as a full time attendant for Brad until he was strong enough to do daily routines and enjoy the time with his family in the house on his own.

Joseph Brown, who was trained as a private aide whom they found through Moses, his nurse at Burke. He worked with Brad every day, hour upon hour— to cover simple to complex tasks, and without a problem, Joseph became an essential member of the family for eight months. When Brad eventually returned home, his sons were overjoyed, and Joseph showed them how to help him in their youthful fashion. He told the boys to keep looking forward and set goals for themselves as to how they could help their father progress.

Said Joseph of Brad's recovery: "Over the time I spent with him and his family, he improved tremendously. His speech since I have known him has always been splendid, his walking has improved, and his arm movement is much better. He is someone who has never given up the opportunity to be his old self and he is always in good spirits. This characteristic sped up his well-being. He smiled, regardless of what is thrown at him and I respect and admire his courage. I am really happy that I was part of his health recovery team."

Today, I am so pleased to see how well and robust Brad looks and he is working full time. Now I am sure that he would get even better because he's a living miracle.

CHAPTER TEN

NO PARENT WANTS to see their child suffer—not even from a bad cold. But Brad's journey through hell was wholly different. His healing took years, but the pieces fell together as one could hope. It started with the first angel, Natalie who saved his life in the ambulance, Then Dr. Mohan took Brad to surgery for the craniotomy. After that procedure was complete, Brad was put into an induced coma for a month, and the whole family watched as he slowly returned to being awake.

From that point on, the hardest work began. Everyone questioned his ability to fully heal, but I knew him better. His recovery was not imminent, but slowly creeping toward a more normal way of life. Brad always had a vision and was very demanding of himself. He helps his community as much as possible and works just as hard every day at his career. What is most interesting is that his advice is always counted on by his friends because he always goes for the gold.

From the beginning, we all took on as much responsibility as we could to ease the load on Jessica. Noah was just beginning Kindergarten, weeks after the stroke. On the first day of school, Jessica, Marsha, and I took him there, without Brad. It was an emotional event for all of us and Noah handled as well as any child could while he was deeply missing his father.

Jessica took him to school every day thereafter and then went to see Brad as, he was guided by the nurses, the physical therapists, and the other professionals through the work that would strengthen his body and mind.

From August 4 on, I kept a watchful eye the people who worked with him, always hoping for regained strength, emotional response, and success in each day's work. I turned to God to show his powers of healing, never knowing what I would see the next day.

But perhaps I was rewarded for my prayers as Brad continued to recover.

It wasn't till weeks into the incident that I found out for sure that he had suffered a stage five stroke … the worst kind which meant he had slim to no chance of survival, but it seems that his age and healthy body had supported all efforts to make him whole again.

Looking back on August 4, 2013, I realized how mind boggling this journey has been. As early as the day before Brad's stroke, I was successfully managing a doctor's office, near where we lived, enjoying our lives. Our children were grown and married, and we were doting grandparents. So we moved to our lovely condo complex less than 20 minutes away and fell in love with our new home.

It took a short time to adapt to our new community and we met a circle of people who had come there to live from all over the tristate area. Less than a year later, the ax fell. I remember that morning so clearly. It was 7:30 am and we had our bags packed to go to the pool in our complex and were headed out the door when our daughter in law called and yelled in the phone,

"Come quickly! Brad is not well!" If ever there was an understatement, that was it. Fortunately, we lived close by and made it to their house before the ambulance left the driveway. Brad was already in the ambulance with Natalie Dawn, the first medical specialist to lay hands on him. We consider Natalie our first savior. She encouraged Brad to breathe and stay awake. But he went into seizures and then fell into unconsciousness.

I remember driving behind the ambulance in a taxi as we followed Brad to the local hospital where he was first taken. But the next few hours were a blur because I do not remember walking into Westchester Medical Center or seeing his doctors and nurses as they prepared him for surgery. Shortly thereafter, Brad's brother-in-law, Dr. Ron Aboody, an interventional radiologist reviewed all the scans and declared that the brain bleed was a grade five AVM or an Atrial Ventricular Malformation. The room was silent as those who considered Brad's projected treatment had virtually nothing to say.

Most doctors would avoid getting involved with this condition, because there was virtually no chance of recuperation. We heard it directly from them in the emergency room and fate seemed to be the answer to our questions. At best, he could be semi-alert, and in a wheelchair for however long he lived.

But Dr. Mohan did save his life when he operated on the Arteriovenous Malformation. That is when the medically induced coma was introduced to his stricken body to heal for a month. There was lots of uncertainty as to whether he would wake up and recover. But after the full month passed, he started to slowly recover. From that day on, they began physical therapy on Brad and every day I visited him.

Each day and every day, I would go to Brad's room on the third floor ICU. It is where Dr. Mohan's patients recovered, and my son was tightly hanging on to his life. Day after day, Dr. Mohan would attempt to wake Brad up by shouting loudly at him to no avail.

Jennifer, his primary nurse, always spent extra time with us. One Thursday, Brad was motionless. Some of the staff felt he was heading downhill, but I never believed that. Jennifer explained that he just needed a restful day, and we took her words seriously.

She was correct. By the following day, his eyes were open and alert.

Then came the move to the Helen Hayes Rehab Facility in Haverstraw, New York and the next phase began.

CHAPTER ELEVEN

WHEN MY SON, Brad suffered the stroke, my first thought was, "how could this happen to him?" What would life be like without my son who Marsha and I raised to be the exceptional man he is?

A piece of my heart was virtually ripped out. When I saw him after his life saving surgery, I was taken aback by the way he looked. His head was both shaved and swollen and we were told that a piece of his skull had been removed. What did they do to my son?

From the very beginning, we all had certain tasks to do to make Jessica's life as easy as possible. That day, Jessica, Marsha, and I took Noah to Kindergarten.

We had to leave him there without his father around to say goodbye. The thought of Noah not having his dad with him, and for a long time to come, if ever, made me cry in public. I walked out of the Murray school in Larchmont—my face full of tears because I was wholly unable to face that scene anymore. For many days thereafter, I would cry all the way to work.

Brad was in a coma for over a month. I went to visit him on every lunch hour since my office was closed at that time. But the day he came out of the coma, I got to see him with his eyes wide open and I was in shock! My boy was coming back! He was able to give me a high five with his right hand and his awareness of everyone around him was back!

Every visit became a joy. By the time he was transferred to the Helen Hayes Rehab center, I actually tested his memory about taxes. After all, he was a tax attorney. While he still had such a long recovery in front of him, he could actually recite sections of the Internal Revenue tax code—incredible!

His most difficult issue became speech and I spent hours each day trying to figure out how to encourage him to speak when he was totally silent. When Brad was still in Helen Hayes, I started to think of ways to encourage him to communicate. One day, I stepped out of his room with my cell phone and decided to call my son on his phone.

I casually said, "Hi Brad" and he said, "Hi Dad," and we had a short conversation.

His speech therapist jumped into the change of the speech and took what was first garbled and incomplete phrases and made them beautifully clear again.

Within months of starting rehab and all the various types of therapies, I knew he was yearning to drive again. Defying his wife's orders, I let him drive around the block in my car. I felt such joy because he became the happiest guy in the world behind the wheel.

Some of the things he enjoyed were no longer available to him. I miss sharing them with him as well. I will always miss our tennis matches together, or football and baseball catches may be gone for good. But seeing Brad thrive is one of the best things that ever happened to me. It encouraged me to remember how he grew to be a person I truly admired, and I knew at that point, he'd be back again.

Shortly after Brad awakened, the doctors advised that we bring the children in to see their father. It was important for them know that he would not look like the vigorous man he once was, but his wasted face and body were still the ones the children adored.

One Sunday morning, Jess and the children arrived at the medical center with breakfast for the family. On the way up to the sixth floor, Noah asked, "Is this what heaven looks like?" All along, he had worried that what he had been told was not true, and that his father had died. While initially hesitant and scared, the boys were quickly overjoyed!

The greeting was uproarious, and the children did not care about the changes everyone else has worried about. They were just overjoyed to have their father alive, getting better, and back in their lives.

From that time forward, they were able to see him on a more regular basis when he was transferred to Helen Hayes Rehab shortly thereafter. There they got to watch the intense work of his physical therapy and how it would slowly improve his body and his mind.

CHAPTER TWELVE

EVERY YEAR, ALMOST **8,000** people in the United States have a stroke. About 610,000 of these are first or new strokes. If they are not treated in time, the chance to live diminishes by the minute. Brad was lucky that day that the stroke took place in his own house and his wife was nearby.

It took over two months of intensive surgery and treatment to lift him to the place where his battered brain and body could continue to heal with the most ingenious mechanics and professionals who know how to treat the patient and use the technology. Was it fundamental teamwork or incredible determination?

Brad was extremely lucky that his employer, General Electric, and his fellow employees were totally supportive of him and it made us all feel more secure in many ways. The Glasgow Coma Scale was administered at least once a day to ensure that Brad was making strides and would be able to stay at the center to continue his journey. That is when his Physical Therapy, Occupational Therapy and Speech Therapy began in earnest. They used a technique called neuroplasticity.

This technique provides the ability for the brain to form and reorganize connections via learning and experiences following an injury. The brain has the ability to reorganize itself by forming new neural connections throughout life. Neuroplasticity allows the neurons (nerve cells) in the brain to compensate for injury and disease and to adjust their activities in response to new situations or changes in their environment given time.

The proportion of gray matter can change, and synapses may strengthen or weaken.

In Brad's case, the practitioners worked to optimize the natural networks after his brain injury. Research in the latter half of the twentieth century indicated many aspects of the brain can be altered even throughout adulthood. This malleable attribute makes a large difference in the brain's ability to recover.

The regular testing of Brad's brain indicated the changes brought about by neuroplasticity. I watched the way his coordinators, Maria, the head nurse on the floor, oversaw all the therapy he endured, and it was tough as she handled his physical workouts. I was overwhelmed with her concentrative precision.

Ronnie was the most nurturing nurse on the floor. She soothed Brad when he had nothing left to give. Ronnie helped Brad with his memory which was spotty and become, over a relatively short period of time, quite cohesive.

They left nothing out and ensured that the times when he would falter would not go unnoticed. I would cry and so would Ronnie who reassured me that even when Brad was weakened by exhaustion, he would rebound under their supervision.

Lindsay, another one of Brad's therapists would play Brad's favorite music for him constantly and that would put a smile on his face. When I was upset, Maria calmed me down. Lindsay and Ronnie would work so hard that tears often came to their eyes as well. All three of the therapists were guardian angels and were a godsend to Brad, Bobby, and me.

It was at Helen Hayes rehab, that Brad was trained to walk again. It was a huge transition for a man who had been prone for so long.

The improvement of motor recovery and neuron plasticity of a patient along specific patterns is the aim of rehabilitation exercises. The use of robotic technology in rehabilitation can accelerate the treatment and recovery of the disabled and it actuates the rehabilitation clinics to change their path from labor-intensive operations to technology-assisted operations.

Later on, when Brad arrived at Burke for extended rehab, emerging robotic technology in a traditional rehabilitation therapy session would provide high quality treatment at a lower cost and effort. The level of motor recovery of patients can be quantified by defining different rehabilitation exercises for the robot.

What makes this so important is that different lower limb rehabilitation-assisting robots have been developed to revive the functional mobility of damaged limbs, ranging from complex computerized stations to simple structures. These systems have been categorized in five different groups:

- Treadmill gait trainers
- Foot-plate-based gait trainers
- Overground gait trainers
- Stationary gait trainers
- Ankle rehabilitation systems.

In some studies, resistive force has been provided during exercise and high flexibility in performing a different range of motions.

To develop the robotic devices, first the motor learning and motor adaption of healthy people has been investigated; and then the neurologically injured patients can be rehabilitated with respect to the obtained results.

Therapeutic exercises can vary from range of motion. The effect of all these opportunities had a growing effect on Brad's healing process.

Healthy participants' data has been used to evaluate the capability of a parallel robot during four various rehabilitation exercises. The performance of the robot based on real patient data during normal walking has been investigated at other rehabilitation sites.

The aim of this study is to investigate and evaluate different characteristics of the parallel robot during the performance of different exercises for the rehabilitation of a lower limb.

Focusing the attention on a single leg, it is composed of two links connected to each other by a cylindrical joint and connected to the top and to the base by two respective universal joints. The improvement of motor recovery and motor plasticity of a patient along specific patterns is the aim of rehabilitation exercises for true success.

The use of robotic technology in rehabilitation can accelerate the treatment and recovery of the disabled and it actuates the rehabilitation clinics to change their path from labor-intensive operations to technology-assisted use. Emerging robotic technology in a traditional rehabilitation therapy session would provide high quality treatment at a lower cost and effort. The level of motor recovery of patients can be quantified by defining different rehabilitation exercises for the robot as more mechanics and methodology are devised and developed over time.

CHAPTER THIRTEEN

"When the Fund Began"

AT THIS TIME, we realized that fundraising for more robotic and exoskeleton availability was a necessity for Brad as well as so many others who would benefit from our efforts. Jess became the brains and effort behind our challenges to bring the ideal mechanics to Burke for Brad's use as well as others who struggled with the same issues.

An Ekso Exoskeleton Gait System produced by Ekso Bionics and the MIT Anklebot Robotic Limb Technology made all the difference. The exoskeleton is a powered light weight soft suit intended for use with lower limb disability due to a stroke. It is the only post-stroke gait training solution that provides systematic gait training throughout the spinal column.

In short, training with the Anklebot, as well as a wearable exoskeleton which provides powered hip and knee motion which enables individual with neuropathic injuries to stand upright, walk turn, climb, and even descend stairs. It made a significant difference in his gait. The full body robotic exoskeleton is the first of its kind to receive FDA clearance for personal and rehabilitation use in the United States.

Brad also used robots produced by the Krebs Lab at MIT which had just been cleared by the FDA. The ankle bot helped him regain dorsiflexion in his left ankle. He also used a wrist robot to regain movement and strength in his left wrist.

Not long ago, this would not have been possible. The relative severity of the injuries would have required only a wheelchair to get around. The exoskeleton is a device you wear on the outside, changed the possible outcomes.

Technically, it is a wearable skeleton. It can be strapped onto and over legs, hips, the torso, and arms. It is not quite a robotic since it does not do all the work for you. This apparatus is not like armor, because it does not remain still, nor does it do all the work for you. These exoskeletons have sensors and power. But it requires the patient's sensors and a tremendous amount of willingness to use his or her own power!

There is plenty that goes into constructing an exoskeleton. It is constructed with petrochemicals which are fiber-reinforced epoxy resin propylene and benzene.

If you do not spend nine to five in a chemical manufacturing lab these names may be unknown to you, but in simpler terms, here is how the construction goes:

From crude oil or natural gas petrochemicals are created. For the exoskeletons, various materials like ABS and polycarbonate are used. From the plastics that come from these chemicals, we can make anything plastic—even exoskeletons!

Physical therapists who teach people how to use the device have more than one story about people who get up, walk across a room for the first time after their injury. Such was the experience for Brad who cried along with his therapist with the knowledge that he was on the road to mobility.

That is not to say that it was easy. After fifteen minutes in the exoskeleton, Brad was sweating bullets. It is a workout like non-other, but for those who believed they never walk again it is an unimaginable gift.

But the fact is that the exoskeleton is not a workout machine. You put one on so that you can walk across the room, but it is the patient who is doing the work. What you learn to do in a relatively short amount of time is that you can walk up and down stairs, walk outside, in a park, on the grass with your friends and loved ones.

Brad specifically used a full body robotic exoskeleton in order to work on his gait. He also used robots produced by the Krebs Lab at MIT. The ankle bot helped him regain dorsiflexion in his left ankle. He also use a wrist robot to regain use of his left hand and wrist.

With this capability and knowledge, and use of these miracle machines, Brad was well on his way back.

CHAPTER FOURTEEN

AFTER SIX WEEKS at Helen Hayes Rehab, Brad was transferred to NYU Langone where he met his next savior, Dr. Riina, whose job it was to transfer the part of Brad's brain, previously lodged in his stomach, back to his skull. Dr. Riina is an expert in many types of neurosurgery.

In addition to providing care, Dr. Riina is active in research and has been involved in developing new devices and treatments for many neurovascular conditions. His most recent work has included the development of new minimally invasive devices to treat brain aneurysms, a tracheal stent to treat vocal cord and airway collapse, as well as intra-arterial chemotherapy for recurrent malignant brain tumors.

"I chose to pursue a career in neurosurgery because I wanted to help people, and I was drawn to patient care and treatment innovation. I enjoy working with people, and as a vascular neurosurgeon, my goal is to educate my patients and make them feel at ease in dealing with complex problems," he added during one of our conversations.

He wanted to know my background and wondered why I was more aware of medical procedures than many of his patients or their families. I told him that I managed a doctor's office for over 25 years and only left because of Brad's plight.

I told him that I did miss talking to the patients in the waiting and examining rooms, but I belonged with Brad. While I watched my son go through his therapy, I would whisper:

"You can have it all; You have my heart. Do not you dare die. The stars are aligned, and you will wake up and become alert. You have your whole life ahead of you. Rest and reach for the rainbows … Count your blessings! You can have it all …"

CHAPTER FIFTEEN

"I FIRST HEARD about Brad in the early morning at my home on Long Beach Island. The news devastated me, said Ron Oboody, a radiological neurologist." My healthy and energetic brother-in-law was unresponsive.

One the way to the Westchester Medical Center, I read reports of his Cat Scan from the small hospital to which he had initially been taken. The report described a probable aggressive hemorrhagic brain tumor. As a neurologist, I knew this would be a death sentence. Then I spoke to his neurosurgeon who assured me that he would remove a large section of Brad's skull to relieve pressure as soon as an MRI was performed.

Upon arriving at the medical center, I was initially relieved to hear that the current diagnosis could potentially be treated.

Our relief was short lived as the MRI showed extensive damage to the brain. All we could do was hope for the best outcome which seemed dim. The comatose period after the initial surgery seemed endless. This was followed by what we called "The Foggy Brain Period," which was even worse. While he learned to speak again, there was a terrifying emptiness to his words. We all sadly entered what we termed, the "Pseudo-Brad Stage."

Gradually, I noticed week to week improvement and finally a shred of hope during my weekly visits to Burke Rehabilitation Center in White Plains. During this time period, he actually started to become Brad again!

Finally his abrasive dry sense of humor returned in full force and I felt a real sense of joy. That is when I knew his second life had truly begun. He was finally back.

CHAPTER SIXTEEN

JESSICA SPENT SLEEPLESS nights worrying and pondering the next steps forward. One day in September, she and I sat in a coffee shop in Larchmont. There was no denial of our devastation. I tried to make small talk that would ease our anxiety, and it hurt so badly that the family was only seeing each other at the hospital at the bedside of her beloved husband. We are private people and there was extraordinarily little to talk about besides Brad. We both cried. Jess was someone that had always looked to help others. I sensed it was hard for her to be the one needing the help. I tried to assure her I was there for her, as others would be, and that she should accept the help.

I felt that talking to Jess this way really helped our relationship because it uplifted both of us. I trusted her because she obviously wanted to share my pain and reduce the incredible pressure that was on both of us.

This is when it became clear to her that Brad needed more than typical rehab and that is when the fundraising began.

The exoskeleton was expensive and not covered by insurance, but scholarships were given to people who needed the help, but their insurance companies did not comply. Our fundraising changed not only Brad's successful use of the robotics, but we as a family were thrilled to help others at Burke rehab as well.

At one event, a woman came up to us and said that her son had not walked in years, and she was beyond amazed to see his rehabilitation reach a whole new level. She cried tears of joy and we joined her. So many others benefitted. Miracles happened before our eyes.

Night and day for weeks on end, Jessica researched neurosurgeons all over the country. Her family is composed of many doctors who helped her with the search. When she spoke to several specialists in various states, all told her that Brad needed surgery.

Fortunately, she found Dr Riina who was in New York City. He thought there was a much better way to handle this injury. Dr Rinna's plan saved Brad from being in a wheelchair for the rest of his life. That is where the Gamma Knife helped preserve his ability to walk and to heal. It was hard to be a young mom, raising two children and having an important job while Brad struggled to make strides in his struggle to be well again. Through all that she did to improve the situation, she also convinced her company to change their insurance policies, and they did so by covering all his expenses. That was a huge overture. It set a new precedent for how her company dealt with their employee's health issues. When someone in your family gets sick, you move forward to create a balance in your life, and Jessica's determination made great strides for everyone in our family. In my mind, it is legendary.

From Jess:

> "My whole life turned upside down on August 4, 2013. Not surprisingly, over the course of the following eight years—and it continues in the present—I have wrestled through the five stages of grief. Our life was perfect; all I could have dreamed of, and I appreciated every moment. It didn't take Brad having a stroke for me to realize how lucky we were. In hindsight, I can see clearly how much changed for all of us. Every single day I tried my best to be the best I could be for Brad's recovery and to reclaim our life together. Eventually that led us to the final stage of grief, which is acceptance, probably the hardest stage. Acceptance meant that we would all be able to live our best life. It meant that all of our efforts to support Brad and his recovery weren't for naught. I found acceptance through a combination of practices:

journal writing, yoga, running, therapy, and a daily practice of reading the serenity prayer: God grant me the Serenity to accept the things I cannot change, Courage to change the things I can, and Wisdom to know the difference."

CHAPTER SEVENTEEN

JESSICA REVEALED TO me that she was a very private person and as much as I knew she wanted to share things, there was extraordinarily little to talk about besides Brad. I cried often and she tried to comfort me, but when I looked up at her there were always tears flowing down her own cheeks, and this is what she said:

"What makes it so hard for me" she said, "is that I am used to being the helper and I have trouble accepting support from others."

The exoskeleton was expensive and not covered by insurance, but scholarships were given to people who needed the help, but their insurance companies did not comply. Our fundraising changed not only Brad's successful use of the robotics, but we as a family were thrilled to help others at Burke rehab as well.

At one event, a woman came up to us and said that her son had not walked in years, and she was beyond amazed to see his rehabilitation reach a whole new level. She cried tears of joy and we joined her. So many others benefitted. Miracles happened before our eyes.

As the children played, I remember my conversations with Jess. Once she said that she always wanted to help people but neither she nor Brad wanted to be the recipients of the kindness. Brad was given a new perspective in his life and as he saw how he could attain personal growth he was inspired and motivated. It was a collaborative effort to get him to a place of strength and endurance.

CHAPTER EIGHTEEN

WHEN MIT BROUGHT the exoskeleton to Burke. It provided a whole new dimension to Brad's rehab.

Dr Rinna saved him from being in a wheelchair for the rest of his life. That is where the Gamma Knife helped preserve his ability to walk and to heal.

But Jessica felt the need to do more, and that is just what she did. When Brad came home, it was then that she created the fundraising and that became her focus for the next year. Jenny Lewis at Burke became her anchor. That was the start of raising almost one million dollars. The community at large, and friends all over the country, participated in all the events. When you create a clinic that enhances people's chances of recovery, it is a major accomplishment.

People also say things happen for a reason. In Brad's case I could not bear to hear that phrase: What happens in your life is not "lucky?" It is persistence and endurance to achieve your goals that Jess sought out constantly to make this happen for Brad and his family. We gain wisdom as we forge ahead and become amazed at how the body heals when the mind is in the right place.

Jess was a non-stop machine who looked for everything and everyone available to help her husband. She looked for a mind and body connection. She sought out how this process affects your mental health.

Many steps followed, including acupuncture, and other modalities developed for him to succeed. Jessica stopped at nothing. She extended herself in every way possible way to secure a means to help him heal.

She grasped for all that was offered to us. We spent endless hours with her, seeking out every possible way to rehab Brad.

When our family was at stake, we stopped at nothing. Nobody gets in your way. Such was the case with Jessica. The children learned valuable lessons that will be with them forever. Brad's regeneration became their life too. At their tender young ages, they learned how you bond together and seek out help. It was a lesson that was critical and stays with them to this very day.

CHAPTER NINETEEN

DAVE: I WAS running on the morning of August 4, 2013. I remember where I was, and I even remember the song I was listening to. A phone call from my dad cut in so I took it since I was just about home. I still remember the conversation. He asked, "what are you doing?" And I replied, "I'm running." He replied, "well stop running." I knew immediately something was wrong.

My dad told me Brad was being taken to the hospital, but he really did not have a clear understanding of what happened. My head started to spin. Of course he told me not to jump in my car or on a plane, not wanting me to worry or travel. There would be no point to do this so soon. What could I do but be in the way? I listen to my father about so many wise things that he tells me, but this was a different situation.

I walked into my house and my wife was there with our twin daughters, only one year old. I told her what was happening. She told me I needed to get on a plane despite what I was told, and I totally agreed. She immediately turned to the phone and booked me a flight to JFK airport. I was so eternally grateful for her swift action, because I could barely function.

I got on the flight, jumped in a cab when I landed, and went straight to the hospital to find my parents and my brother's wife and her parents.

At that point, I was just relieved that Brad was still alive, and I could be there with them. He had undergone emergency brain surgery of what type I did not know.

When it came time, I went into the room with my parents to see him.

Literally, it was the worst moment of my life. Seeing him like that was overwhelming. He was almost unrecognizable. My big brother: My rock throughout my life was my role model and source of a lot of my strength. Yet now he was unrecognizable. It was truly a nightmare. Without hesitation, I cracked and crumpled to the floor in tears.

Despite the fear, I never doubted Brad's potential to survive because I knew he would never quit. I knew he was otherwise healthy and fit and that if anyone could recover from this, it was he.

And he did miraculous things. Over time, he woke up and recalled old memories with me. He also began to talk. Then he began to walk. He began to crack jokes and laugh. I was inspired like never before in my life or ever expect to in the future.

CHAPTER TWENTY

BRAD'S BEST FRIEND Jake Raddok: I remember when I first heard about Brad's brain hemorrhage. I was on the beach with my family and I got a voicemail from Dave. I actually still have that voicemail. That is when I called Dave back and got the full story, I was totally shocked—maybe in shock too—and incredibly sad. In addition to being one of my best friends, I did not know what to do at the moment.

When I visited him in the hospital the following day, I found him in a medically induced coma and out of reach, I was afraid that the next time I saw him, he would be dead. That was the most terrifying aspect of it all—not knowing if he would wake himself up. The doctors who cared for him seemed quite certain that people in this state do not wake up from comas better than they were before, so the best thing we could hope for was that Brad would wake up at all.

I remember one conversation I had with Brad's dad while in the hospital. Bob worried about how Brad would function—even at a low level.

"What would be the point of life," Bobby sadly wondered.

The recovery was tough to watch. Seeing your buddy relearn to walk, talk, and even breathe was not easy. Now that I reflect on that time, it is a lucky feeling I have, that the stroke may have taken some physical things, but nothing mental agility. Nowadays, Brad and I still have the same things to laugh about and he maintained his same ridiculous sense of humor, I am grateful for all that came back. It was amazing.

Our friendship really has not changed. He is still the guy I turn to when I need a good laugh or a break from reality. I hope I am that for him.

I know that the stroke probably changed some of his relationships, but not ours. I do not feel sorry for him. I do feel sad that it happened in the first place, because I know he would kill to go for a run. But he has a great family, two terrific kids and that is what really matters.

CHAPTER TWENTY-ONE

VANESSA: BRAD ALWAYS was sweet, funny, and incredibly smart. He could before and even now make Dave laugh like no one else. I have always admired their relationship and adore Brad as a brother-in-law and that is why the four of us took a trip to Peru in 2006 together shortly after both Brad and Jess and Dave and I were married and not yet parents.

I never forgot how grateful I am that the stroke did not strike Brad while we were hiking on remote Inca trails. I am wholly certain he would not have survived.

When the stroke did hit, however, it seemed like time stopped. Dave got on the first flight out of Vermont to New York, and I stayed home with our five-year-old and 14-month-old twin daughters. It was terrible not to be able to go with Dave, knowing that no matter what happened with Brad, Dave was about to face the hardest thing yet in his life, and I could not be there to support him, Jess, our parents, and the rest of the family.

Jess rallied friends, the community, colleagues, and friends to be certain that he got the best care possible. She spent a great deal of time seeing that Noah and Andrew's physical and mental wellbeing were taken care of by all the family and friends that cared about them.

CHAPTER TWENTY-TWO

JESSICA'S PARENTS: "FROM the first time we met Brad, we knew he was special," said Phyllis and Ted Cohen, Brad's former in-laws. "He impressed us with his intellect and his ability to connect as well as his kind face.

"Brad was strong, determined and open to new experiences. I remember filming him on a trapeze on the west side in New York City. It was shortly thereafter he met Jessica, that she invited him to join her. I watched Brad fearlessly climb up the ladder, execute a perfectly prompted routine and let go of the trapeze bark doing a somersault onto the net below!

"Upon achieving that feat, he climbed down off the net and said, 'That's it! I did it and I am not doing it again!'

"But Brad was always open to doing new things. When we first met, he had not been impressed with fixing things, yet under my husband Ted's tutelage, he began working on all kinds of projects. When a new piece of furniture required assembly, he even welcomed it as a challenge.

"What I enjoyed the most about him was that he was open to seeing the world from other people's perspective.

"I remember the most beautiful fourth of July weekend that we all spent on Long Beach Island in 2013, a month prior to the stroke. We had taken the boat to a remote private beach near Barnegat Inlet. The weather was perfect, and the water was calm. We were wading in shallow water and the kids were search for some fish and snails. I recall saying that I wished we could stop the clock and never let that moment go. But we all know that is not how life is.

"One month later to the day, we got that fateful call from Jessica. We dropped everything and met her and the rest of the family at Westchester Medical Center. We all prayed day and night that Brad would survive and thankfully he did. It was a team effort as we all banded together with Brad and ensure the wellbeing of Jess and the kids.

"As Brad began his difficult journey to return to us, he never gave up no matter how hard it was for him. Believe me, it was not easy for anyone to stand by and watch as he struggled to get back on his feet.

"I hate to say this, but I never imagined that Brad would be able to live independently and function at a level beyond most people. But he actually, over time, surpassed the level of everyone assumed. This is due to his tenacity, strength, and stubbornness but most of all because of his motivation. And let us not forget the doctors that Jessica and Dave chose to care for him.

"We all feel incredibly proud of Brad and we recognize the challenges he faced along his difficult journey. Now we pray for the continued good health, peace and contentment for everyone else in their loving family."

CHAPTER TWENTY-THREE

LAURA LIPTON, VANESSA'S mother says: On August 4, 2013, my husband Michael and I were relaxing at our home in Burlington, Vermont, when we got a call that was a shock for us and shook the world or so many of our loved ones, particularly my son in law, Dave. His brother Brad had been rushed to the hospital and was in an induced coma following emergency brain surgery. It was so hard to get our heads around the idea that this vital, fit young man who was training to run yet another marathon could possibly be in critical condition.

And so the family rallied, and support systems kicked into full gear and we all held our breath and each other's hands as we waited for Brad to awaken.

But by Memorial Day on the weekend of 2014, Brad and his family visited Vermont. It was a bittersweet time. In years past, that weekend centered around the Burlington Marathon. Members of the family were either entering the race or cheering for the runners. Over the weekend, Michael and Brad chatted over beer and burgers. As I watched them, I could almost see their life's ups and downs—Brad's rising and Michael was in decline. Yet bittersweet joy, hope, pride, and love conquered what had initially seemed like insurmountable obstacles for Brad. Fear, sadness, and pain surrounded Michael as he slowly succumbed to the challenges of his illness.

Now, eight years later have passed. Brad who was once told he would never walk, drive, or work again, is skiing, parasailing, and commuting daily to the international accounting firm in which he specializes in tax law. His independence is a testament to his strength, humility, humor, and constant gratitude.

CHAPTER TWENTY-FOUR

BRAD'S FRIENDS:

Corin Loguidice: almost 30 years ago at Yorktown High School, sitting by the tennis courts I met my best friend. Even after all these years, Berman has stuck by me through thick and thin and always a trusted companion. He is smart, kind and just an all-around great guy. When Berman got sick and I would visit him in rehab, it amazed me to see him go from someone who thought I was my mom, to getting home and now being stronger and more resilient than ever before. He truly is an inspiration to everyone that comes in contact with him. He has an amazing outlook on life and never complains about what he has been through. I'm so thankful to have him as part of my life and so glad he is doing better than ever!

***

Kerry Quellette: I remember meeting Brad when I was in high school. He is a great friend to my sister and someone who always had a smile on his face and always ready to crack a joke. He is a dependable person; someone you could always count on and smart. He was fun to hang out with when we were kids, and I remember spending a lot of time with him.

Whether it was my house, his house or the tennis courts, Brad was and still is an amazing person. Knowing everything that Brad has been through has not changed my perception of him. In actuality, he has amazed me even more as an adult. Still smart, still smiles and still cracks jokes all the time.

He looks on the bright side of things and genuinely cares about everyone else still putting himself last. He is the true definition of perseverance and persistence. I have always been proud to call Brad my friend but I'm even more proud of who he is now!

***

Rosanna Federico: When I found out that Brad experienced an AVM that put him into a coma l, I first questioned, "this happened to my Brad"? I couldn't fathom in that moment that this could possibly happen to him. Brad was healthy, active, and athletic. He had a family. He had a successful life. I went immediately into a panic questioning if he had a chance to survive. I went into a state of shock and disbelief and all I could do in those few minutes was cry and pray. All I wanted to do is see him.

I did get to visit him as soon as he woke up and was allowed visitors. Now, after all this time, I'm so grateful for his recovery, his family, his doctors, and his determination. He is a warrior!

CHAPTER TWENTY-FIVE

IN APRIL 2014, Bobby and I took Brad and Jessica to the Kittle House Restaurant in Chappaqua for a birthday lunch. I wanted the four of us to be alone. We had been lovingly surrounded after going through so much, that it seemed fitting that we went to our favorite restaurant for peace and tranquility.

At first, when we dined, I thought that Brad was a bit quiet and clearly not himself. Regretfully I did not say anything. After all, it had been months since the first signs of an AVM, last August. Jessica noticed a definite change however, and she insisted that we should bring him to NYU Langone for a C-T scan.

Dr. Riina says that AVMs usually take many more treatments and approximately five years to disappear, but by July of 214, Brad had his last Gamma Knife procedure which he required on that April day. The C-T scans that followed indicated that the AVM completely disappeared and showed that the progress made with the last Gamma Knife procedure was permanent.

CHAPTER TWENTY-SIX

2015: AND WE swiftly moved forward. We all wanted to learn how to fundraise all the more, for the magical ways that helped Brad recover as well and as quickly as possible.

I started to question how I could give back to society in some respect. The first place that entered my mind was Northern Westchester Hospital in Mount Kisco, New York. It was there that I was interviewed by a social worker who was the director of the Ken Hamilton Caregivers Center. She counseled me and told me that if you had a tragedy in your family, you might want to distance yourself from that type of volunteer job which was called a caregiver coach. Clearly, she was talking to someone who could relate to her words.

But I was determined to make a difference in this world and insisted that I could and would make the kind of counselor that could help others get through what I had already managed to do.

Despite her misgivings she recognized my determination and gave me a position as a caregiver coach at the hospital, which I loved to do from day one. But as time went on and Brad continued to struggle to be fully whole again, I ultimately realized that I was experiencing symptoms of Post Traumatic Syndrome Disorder.

From time to time, whenever I saw stroke victims at the hospital, my heart pounded out of my chest and I became weak and weepy. After my primary care doctor examined me thoroughly, he said it was not a part of my heart that acted up; it was more like a broken heart.

After months of denial, at the very same time of my weakest moment, one of our good friends who is my age, suffered a stroke and it was harrowing to watch him go through much of what Brad had endured.

That's when I had to admit that I was not as emotionally capable of handling his or everyone else's illness until I healed myself. Regretfully, I had to leave the new job. But after Brad got home, and we all recognized how superbly he had healed, I went back to Burke and talked to Allison and Colleen, the two social workers at Burke who helped me deal with my own issues. They prepared me to deal with it all, over time, and from the start of my therapy I began to feel better.

As I said goodbye to these special people, we walked the campus of Burke and discussed the idea of an actual Caregiver's Center on site. At that moment in time, they recognized the value of such an enterprise, and took my idea to the directors of Burke. Three months later, they started to build a Caregiver Center at Burke. It was the first time that a rehab center developed a resource like that and for once after all that happened to Brad and the family, I was glad I knew what was indeed necessary in all rehab centers and I was so happy I was in on it from the start!

My dream, these days is to be peaceful. When I wake up in the morning, I clear my head by meditating. I fill my lungs with fresh air and commit my intentions and my responsibilities to that day.

I live in a wonderful community and I am devoted and dedicated to my family and friends. I have learned over all this time that flexibility and creativity are a part of this world.

In the spring of 2021, I will start a master's course in psychology and pray that in a few years, I'll be able to add hope to others who have been through tough times as we have. I accept joy in my home no matter in what order it comes in.

CHAPTER TWENTY-SEVEN

MARSHA: BRAD'S INITIAL strengthening progress began at Helen Hayes but progressed at Burke. There he had access to upper body robotics, but the hospital did not have access to the lower body robotic technology. Jessica asked why and learned that the facility lacked the $600,000 needed to acquire them. When we heard about the limited numbers of these technology-assisted devices, we wanted Brad to get the best treatment available here in Westchester NY. That is when we started fund raising for more of these robots that could help other stroke disabled people, as well as Brad.

Jess expected it would take years to raise that amount but with her efforts and enterprise, we were able to raise almost $800,000 to buy the equipment and more helpful assets that made all the difference. Brad was an inpatient at Burke for six weeks—much longer than most rehabilitating patients.

Our first attempt at fundraising was in March of 2014, in Scarsdale at a place called Barry's Gym. At that time, it had a different name. The turnout was endless and there were two rooms allocated to us. One had a flywheel where participants rode specialty bicycles and there is an instructor who donated his time. It was thoroughly inclusive, and we were thrilled at the kindness of those who gave their time without question. Many people from Burke attended as well as friends and family. Food was also donated by a large number of people.

In March, we went to Manhattan Beach, California, and rented a huge house where all of us could stay with a nanny to help out with the children.

We planned an event similar to what we had done in Scarsdale, hosted by Jessica's cousin Eve.

That year we also had children's events in various places. One took place in Larchmont where a teacher played music for the children to sing and dance to and many of Noah and Andrew's friends participated.

Later on that spring, we again arranged races in Flint Park in Larchmont, and both children and adults ran races where fundraising was even more successful. Tee shirts that featured the logo, "Run for Brad" were sold. Later on the tee shirts we sold were changed to "Train for the Brain," as the evolution of his progress changed.

In September of that year, Jenny Lewis of Burke, who was a dynamo, came to Noah's school and set up tables and chairs where the children received information about upcoming events. Lots of information was also shared with them about the brain and we were all surprised at how interested they were in learning how the brain actually works.

There were many more events that taught children how communities come together to support the people who live and work there. We were shocked at the success of our endeavors. One that our community could appreciate fully was called the New Rochelle Mile, where he walked a mile and we had stations set up for fundraising and some included demonstrations of how the brain works for the children to learn. It was a hot summer day but that did not deflect people from participating to the full extent.

Many of Brad's and Jess's friends walked that day and Noah and Andrew walked beside them.

The next huge event was at the Harrison Tennis Club which Jenny Lewis arranged. Food was donated and we worked hard the evening beforehand so that friends could come to play tennis, socialize, and purchase raffle tickets. The items that Jess collected for the event were expensive and inexpensive so that those who participated were able to donate what they felt comfortable spending on tickets.

Next. we arranged a silent auction which was a huge success. Jess had been able to gather valuable new items and memorabilia from those she knew in the field of sports.

We also were surprised and grateful to the clothing and equipment store, J. Crew, when they offered to donate 30 percent of the income from of one day, from their many stores all over the country. I was in the White Plains store; Jess was in Manhattan and many of our friends were in other J Crew stores in different parts of the country.

That fundraising event was one of the most successful of all. During this terrible downtrend due to the Covid-19 virus, we can no longer shop there and in out hearts we continue to thank them in that way for what they did for us.

One day at Burke, when we hosted a race, a woman came over to Jessica and me to thank us because her son had not been able to stand up in years. It was thrilling to hear that the equipment we were able to enable her son to walk and helped many others as well.

There were many other gatherings like the one in the California Pizza Kitchen nearby, where Noah had his birthday, and even more money was raised. The last event that I recall was the most thrilling. Brad walked two miles up a hill, and when he returned to us, we gathered in a huge pack to rejoice at his success!

Brad's children were also frequent visitors to Burke and often made friends with the other patients. One patient suffered a brain hemorrhage after falling and hitting his head while getting out of bed and Noah decided he wanted to fund raise for him so he could get the same treatment as his Daddy. He indeed fulfilled his wish by asking everyone who was invited to his birthday to donate money for this particular patient to receive robotic treatment. Noah actually raised $5000 which would secure over six weeks of robotic therapy for his new friend.

Mission accomplished.

Dr. Riina recalls an email from one of us that he received when Brad began to use the robotics. It showed Brad first move of his left foot toes.

"From that point on I knew he'd been on his feet walking miles in short order." Dr. Riina replied. "There are few people you meet in life like the members of this family and I don't put anything by the Bermans. Nothing is off the table."

And that is how Brad's success occurred. Brad never liked to be doted on, but on that day, he learned to accept it. I am still amazed at how communities come together to support people in need, and it made me happier that we were the ones who gave what was needed most.

To this day, I still imagine a young woman like Jessica, with two young boys and a sick husband facing such a horrific event. What made everything worthwhile in the end is that it becomes clear to us that stroke victims need more than typical rehab and so that is why the fundraising began.

Our fundraising efforts, overall, permitted us to experience something terrific for adults as well as children in the way life can throw you curves and yet let you come out on top.

CHAPTER TWENTY-EIGHT

TO THIS DAY, Brad requires routine imaging of different forms to see inside of his brain. He is the quintessential example of strength and endurance. He wakes up every morning with intention in mind and is eternally grateful for simple things that occur in his life. We, as the members of his family, realized that routine is essential. Brad learned from his own experience that it is quintessential, and his family has learned more, during this period of time, than any other time in our lives.

His emphasis these days is balancing the work he loves with his children who are critically important to him. His voice gives hope to many. As his journey continues, he embraces every opportunity and as a result, he learned his foresight and limitations. What I, as his mother, am most astounded by is how he reconnects with compassion and broadens his circle on a daily basis in order to help others.

Afterall, the normal brain is only a three-pound snarl of tissue. Yet it creates an impressive invention and helps to give us a sense of self.

Brad also learned that silence teaches you about yourself and sleep significantly affects your emotions. When you combine silence, communication, and sleep into a wholesome package you produce a stable person. Brad's recovery required a team approach that adhered to this process.

. We also learned that recovery in the brain is measured in weeks, not months. Much improvement can show up in short integers and is apparent when it slows down later in life. Brad's brain tissue recovered in stages as we found out by what was perceived at Westchester Medical Center are later on by New York Langone Hospital.

All the doctors with whom we are in touch are amazed by the plateaus and stages he reached, and each has said it fulfills their own wishes for all the members of society that they treat.

What they say now is that Brad could or should have lost his life so easily, but some techniques work well for one person and not another, but they use all the compensatory ways of helping each patient.

The caregivers are also part of a successful strategy. We found that out when Brad came home and was treated by a host of physical therapists and support staff who made the difference. Those who worked with him established routines and included daily tasks. They encouraged him to write notes for himself in his memory book.

As a member of our "tag team," I started journaling that August and continued thereafter. I remember one day when I took some time away, that I got a call from the Helen Hayes Rehab that Brad had fallen from a platform. From that day forward, I knew I had to be there with him, at Westchester Medical, Helen Hayes, Langone and Burke and anywhere else he still needed me.

During this period, I was distracted and had trouble making decisions and had to distance myself from my friends because I needed to be a private person at that time.

Finally, Brad arrived home in December 2013, where he was greeted by all of us with a special congratulatory dinner. We were all overwhelmed when we personally reviewed how far he had come. For months thereafter, Brad became an outpatient at Burke to continue his therapy, four days a week.

But Jessica had come a long way too. She arranged to have metal bars placed along the walls throughout the house and in the bathrooms so Brad could safely bathe and traverse their home with ease. She worked at not overworking him but guiding him in a manner that his ultimate success was placed on a circle of people—not just one.

Jonathan Mroz, a physical therapist also at Burke, vividly remembered the first time he met Brad when he was an outpatient at the center.

"It was a cold late fall afternoon in late fall and Brad was my last patient of the day. Brad arrived with his wife for his initial evaluation. I already knew a little bit about him after speaking to my supervisor as well as

Andrea from the in-patient department. Charts and all the documentation that had been collected regarding his convalescence. I remember he and Jessica were visibly engaged in the session and said they were eager to try anything and everything to help Brad get better.

"Since I did not know him yet, I was not aware of it but looking back, I think he was a little nervous and unsure about how much he would be able to recover. I also recall that he did not speak that much on the first day but now I realized that this was unusual for him. It was encouraging to see that Jessica was so supportive as I worked with him over the next two years and saw how amazing his support system really was.

"I also got to see how determined, competitive, and ambitious he is. All of these attributes served him well on his road to recovery and beyond.

"Although his health condition was extremely complicated, and there were specific medical guidelines that were set by the surgeon, what he could or could not initially do, I was confident, based on Brad and Jessica's attitude and eagerness to learn, that he would regain as much of his prior abilities as possible.

"It was a great pleasure to work with him and I am proud of how much he accomplished. I always set high goals for my patients however, Brad surely surpassed the expectations I had for him when I met him that first day."

Of all the finest nurses who cared for Brad while at Burke was a man named Moses. When he was not there, I was disappointed and disturbed. My tolerance in some of the other professional's lackadaisical manner put me at an all-time low. As his mother, I think that is when my original behavior of kindness and support for others substantially changed. Fortunately, when Brad made dramatic transformation in his healing, I started to return to my usual behavior.

My approach to people now is more open and I have a special place in my heart for those who need help. To this day, I am eternally grateful that the right doctors where chosen to change the direction of his condition. For a long time, I had continuous nightmares and I feared the phone ringing in the middle of the night. I calmed my fears by calling the hospital every day when I was there even though I arrived there every morning. I was constantly afraid of what I would see or learn once I arrived there.

Now I do not feel overwhelmed, but instead, I am overjoyed, and I breathe easily because the best outcomes result from a clear head and compassionate approach. It is interesting to me that as a result of Brad's catastrophe, I feel more sensitivity and my love continues to grow. I have grown and moved forward from inside out.

Another thing I learned by surprise is that laughter is a healing way to respond to frustration and exhaustion. We feel relieved and renewed when we share humor. There is a balance between laughter and compassion. We look to others this way through their insights.

Listening and sharing are part of recovery for the patient and family alike. It sustains the caregiver's strength to bounce off of other people. I found that this mechanism helped me feel calmer and more peaceful. This way, we create meaningful connections and consider all our opportunities to enhance our lives to the fullest when we replenish our souls. I found balance this way.

During this time, I became a relentless researcher. I read everything I could about Brad's AVM and even read medical journals about the condition and learned a tremendous amount I never heard about before. In order to help him and understand everything his doctors told us; I knew I needed to educate myself on the subject. My goal was not to let anything get in my way as we went through this experience. As I healed along with my son, I grabbed whatever happiness I could, otherwise there would come a point where I would run out of time.

After a short time of my demands for my son, staff members would see me appear and knew I would not tolerate ineffective assistance. But Moses was as efficient as any member of the group could be and I enjoyed bringing him breakfast in the mornings when he was too busy to eat.

CHAPTER TWENTY-NINE

AT THE END of Brad's stay in the Westchester Medical Center, I apologized for my behavior to all who had treated Brad. But as a mother, I recognized that every step of the way was critical, and I had insisted on that fact.

We can forgive what feels untenable when we learn that we benefit the most by letting go and moving on. I also learned not to fight for closure, not to choose answers and not expect everyone to understand. Inner peace is critical, and it is imperative to learn not to respond in a negative manner to everything that bothers you. I almost felt like I had gone back to college with the knowledge that was imbued on me by everyone who connected with us at each of the hospitals.

We all needed support to get through this disaster and support groups are critical to have on the wellness team. A brain injury is traumatic to every member of the family and bearable only through perseverance. It always requires balancing homelife, therapy of all kinds and plans to work again.

At this point in the healing process, the patient must learn relaxation technique and remember to use or develop a sense of humor. Brain injury, after all, may affect vision perception and clear thinking. Returning to work requires successful therapy to improve or succeed in relinquishing these problems.

What makes our family happiest is that Brad has become a superb mentor to so many men and women who have experienced brain bleeds. It was great to watch him intentionally conceptualize ideas to help others.

It was quite difficult for a private person like Brad to put himself out there and offer important information to those who need help with the overwhelming issues.

Everyone with brain bleeds of all kinds are looking for answers. This work helped him return to being the great dad, an active participant in society and getting back to a work-related experience.

When Brad was able to work at his computer again, he joined The AVM Survivor's Network, run by a man named Ben. His last name remains anonymous as do the names of the other members of the group, The network provides peer to peer support between people from all over the world who have dealt with AVM. New members. are welcomed and guided through the site with videos and stories of the members who share information, treatment symptoms and side effects, along with the opportunity to introduce themselves and share their story about AVM. Included on this site are resources written by members for member and notes from the moderators who are long standing member of the site. They strongly encourage all members to explore the pages and the ever-growing information found on these pages.

The mission at Ben's Friends, the colloquial name for the network, is to ensure that patients living with rare diseases or chronic illnesses, as well as their caregivers, family, and friends, have a safe and supportive place to connect with others like themselves.

If you join, you would be asked to start a discussion with your story, thereby answering questions and discussing the practical aspects of dealing with an AVM. Discussions run from the beginning of therapy to learning about how to find affordable medical and fighting health insurance companies.

Feeling down? Need to rant? This is the place to share it all.

This is also the place to discuss all the healing modalities that help the patients cope with AVM which nourishes the mind, body, and spirit. They are asked to discuss any new therapies they are trying with their physician.

In addition, there is the latest worldwide news regarding treatment and success stories that are included in a blog fashion. This part of the site includes discussion about the site itself, its organization, how it works and how it can be improved—just like the needs of those who have been struck by AVM itself.

Feedback and photos are also requested by other members who read the stories and comment or commiserate.

CHAPTER THIRTY

DIANA CASTALDINI WAS first introduced to Brad in the Facebook support group for those who endured and survived an AVM.

"I had just been told that my AVM was incompletely obliterated by the Gamma Knife radiosurgery that I received, which is medical speak for 'not gone yet.'" He commented on a post I wrote because he received the same procedure and we exchanged phone numbers as people often do when they share a medical condition.

Being the compassionate, caring person he is, he sensed that I needed support, so he checked on me frequently via text and phone. This communication quickly led us to develop a friendship.

I soon learned of Brad's recovery journey that had been featured in the media. My first thoughts upon watching the clips were how utterly remarkable this man was to have suffered so greatly—to have lost so much and to be so determined to reclaim his life—all without an ounce of bitterness.

I was deeply moved by his courage, inspired by his strength, and awed by the progress he had made since his stroke. I also noticed how handsome he was and what a beautiful family he had. I felt blessed to have connected with him.

About a year later, after sustaining a friendship on the phone, Brad and I met for the first time. To say I was nervous was an understatement! We sat down and talked for an hour or two about our medical histories and showed each other our scars. We felt calm and at peace just being next to each other—much like kindred spirits.

I was impressed by how well he walked despite his injury on the left side, but even more than that, I was impressed with his tenacity, wisdom, and optimism.

Soon after that, we began dating and we have been together ever since. I extremely lucky to be with my best friend.

Brad also shared his stories and concern for others, especially Heidi Spitz, who was a psychologist at Burke, mentored Brad in a workshop style group of those who had had similar injuries to the brain. It was then that Brad's memory came back through playing games with the boys reading to them and choosing books for himself. But the best choice he made was to go back to work from home until he was strong enough to work full time at his office. His days were full time for the family, work at his office and physical therapy that he did with a specialist at the end of each day. The last thing he thinks about is to be kind and rewind.

What I learned from his routine was that when your child—at any age—is sick, your own mental health suffers. Changes come slowly and that process for me is and ongoing process. I continue to surround myself with people that support and encourage my own efforts to steer my life in the direction I want it to go. I am aligning myself with my own mission, not an intermission.

CHAPTER THIRTY-ONE

JUNE OF THAT year was particularly meaningful. It was filled with all types of events for the cause. The most fun was the run in Flint park. But long before we were able to see the mastery of Brad's efforts, he and Jess were recognized for the yearly Burke Award in 2015.

Senator Kristen Gillebrand also sent a video of praise for the widespread efforts our family and friends made to be of help to others.

On this occasion, Burke was celebrating its one hundred years of service to the Westchester community and beyond.

In addition, the funding provided a rare research organization to conduct ongoing studies to aid the brain injured population and added to the number of neurological scientists to join the faculty at Weill Cornell Medical College in New York City.

Years have passed since that awful day in 2013 Brad is back to being a fun-loving dad to Noah and Andrew as he focuses on his career as well. Each day he says he is grateful to be alive.

Brad is still sweet, funny, and smart and I am so thankful to have him in our lives and proud of my family for moving forward with fundraising to make rehabilitation faster and better for others.

I must admit that I have learned a lot from my son. Every doctor that treated him, but one, thought he would surely die. But we all saw something in him that we believed was different from their initial diagnosis. He had the endurance to live and every day is dedicated to the care of his family.

There is no challenge that Brad will not try to achieve and ultimately make it succeed. He shows his boys every day, how to be a better person.

In fact, with trepidation, I watched him relearn how to drive with the help of Burke's professionals. It was joy to see him take himself back and forth from physical therapy and to work as well.

We would not have endured this challenge nearly as well without the support of our community. Everyone was so impressive and dedicated as well as instrumental in taking care of our family. People have their own hardships but some communities band together to help each other. Teamwork is critical. It was so heartwarming to see these people come together. There are still so many unanswered questions, but we seek the answers on a regular basis. The question has always been and always will be: Why did this happen to Brad?

CHAPTER THIRTY-TWO

STAIRS: THEY SCARED me silly and that is when the hardest work began. Brad literally began to climb the stairs to success. The therapists taught me how to help him when they were not there by standing in front of him on the steps. It gave him security.

That memory is still so strong in my mind because once he fell while walking the stairs with me. We both could have slipped down the stairway not knowing what would happen next. It was an exhausting experience for both of us, but it proved to him in gentle ways that he was on his way back when he got up and finished the climb. Ultimately, he developed a better perception of himself and his future.

On August 4, 2014, we had a party to celebrate one year since Brad's stroke. We called the occasion, "Take Back the Fourth." About 50 people—friends, family and those who helped him progress attended, and Brad, Jess and Noah spoke of their joy and admiration for Brad.

As a team—doctors, physical therapists and friends alike made Brad capable of relearning all that he had lost. His father faithfully rode with him in Brad's car as he gained increasing confidence on the road.

Our nanny for the boys was Valrie whom we needed as much as any supplier or support for a family. We developed a love for he as she did for us, and she kindly kept the boys engaged in activity so that they could put aside the fear they had about their father. It was a time to balance feelings and together, they managed to superbly do a masterful job. The boys learned that life does not go in a straight line. There are always curves in the road. Their support was something we all needed, and all of those we relied upon, supplied more than their share.

To this day, Brad works out remotely over Zoom.us with Andre Lundy, a highly respected physical trainer, to tone his muscles and increase his skills. He still copes with a mild limp in his left leg and a somewhat weak left arm. Yet he is determined to return those small issues to normal once again.

"Brad and I started working together over four years ago," said Lundy. "I was selected to work with Brad due to my pre- and post-rehabilitation certification, and my exercise therapy background. During this lengthy stretch of time, Brad has made significant improvements in his gross and fine motor skill development, functional movement, and overall core and fully body strength. The physical improvements are nothing short of amazing and inspiring to many. I always look forward to our training and pushing to the limits on what is possible.

"During this span of time, Brad has made significant improvement in his gross and fine motor skills development, functional movement and overall core and full body strength. Brad's physical improvements are nothing short of amazing and inspiring to many. I look forward to our continued training and pushing the limits of what is possible."

CHAPTER THIRTY-THREE

ANDREA SULLIVAN WHO was Brad's occupational therapist at Burke said, "When Brad came in for his routine evaluation, I immediately recognized the amount of love and support he had from his family. Throughout his recovery, he was positive and committed to improving physically, functionally, and emotionally, as well. We worked on movement in his arm and hand, but also addressed the independence Brad needed and wanted to resume his life. Independence is critical to anyone who is stricken with a condition that reduces or removes the ability to be normally functional. It faced Brad in a big way and although we wanted to help him thrive, there was much that he needed to do by himself.

"Brad became more independent with basic self-care activities and progressed to returning and driving over the course of his therapy. He arrived with a smile on his face every day and never complained. His attitude helped so many other patients stay positive and get strength to continue to work hard through him. Encouragement to others was a treasured characteristic. Brad taught not only the other patients about recovery, but the staff as well. I am happy to say I am in touch with him regularly and I am amazed at what he has been able to achieve given where he started in his journey."

Without the help of physical, occupational and speech therapists, Brad would not have progressed with the vigor and finesse that he shows today. Among those who helped outside the hospitals were: Andrea and Jonathan. We will never forget them or stop thanking them in our hearts.

On the other hand, there were those who did not help as much as they could. One physical therapist spend most of her time training an intern and not doing her job. I watched her ignore Brad for a while and then went to the director of Physical Therapy and explained that my son was not the person to be trained in how to do the job.

Things changed immediately and when other people did not do their job as expected, I responded in the same manner. I even surprised myself with my change in attitude. Unlike me, Brad learned quickly to let things roll off his back and look forward to his success. But it was my responsibility to become that involved and proceed with my goals for his recovery.

Listening and sharing are part of recovery for the patient and family alike. It sustains the caregiver's strength to bounce off of other people. I found that this mechanism helped me feel calmer and more peaceful. This way, we create meaningful connections and consider all our opportunities to enhance our lives to the fullest when we replenish our souls. I found balance this way.

After a short time of my demands for my son, staff would see me appear and knew I would not tolerate ineffective assistance. But Moses was as efficient as any member of the staff could possibly be.

At the end of his stay in the Westchester Medical Center, I apologized for my behavior, but as a mother, I recognized that every step of the way was critical, and I had insisted on that fact.

We can forgive what feels untenable when we learn that we benefit the most by letting go and moving on. I also learned not to fight for closure, do not choose answers and do not expect everyone to understand. Your inner peace is critical, and it is imperative to learn not to respond in a negative manner to everything that bothers you. It serves no one involved with a "dust up."

We all needed support to get through this disaster and support groups are critical to have on the wellness team. A brain injury is traumatic to every member of the family and bearable through perseverance. It always requires balancing homelife, therapy of all kinds and plans to work again.

At this point in the healing process, the patient must learn relaxation technique and remember to use or develop a sense of humor. Brain injury, after all, may affect vision perception and clear thinking.

Returning to work requires successful therapy to improve or succeed in removing these problems.

What makes our family happiest is that Brad has become a superb mentor to so many men and women who have experienced brain bleeds. It was remarkable to watch him intentionally conceptualize ideas to help others. It was quite difficult for a private person like Brad to put himself out there and offer important information to those who need help with the overwhelming issues.

Everyone with brain bleeds of all kinds are looking for answers. This work helped him return to being the great dad, an active participant in society and getting back to a work-related experience.

Life is better these days despite the lengthy Covid-19 pandemic. Support from family all the way through has been an unwavering effort and we all believe it made the difference.

CHAPTER THIRTY-FOUR

JUNE OF 2015 was particularly meaningful. It was filled with all types of events for the cause. The most fun was the run in Flint park. But long before we were able to see the mastery of Brad's efforts, he and Jess were recognized for the yearly Burke Award in 2015. On Tuesday, June 10 he was presented with a trophy by Josh Berman, the CNN co-anchor of the morning show for his mentorship of so many others he advised and supported along the way.

On this occasion, Burke was celebrating its one hundred years of service to the Westchester community and beyond.

John Matheson Burke, a New York philanthropist has advised those who will handle his estate to provide progressive convalescent care for those who have been released from hospitals but are not well enough to return home. His request was that the funding would provide a facility which would be named for his mother, Winifred Masterson Burke.

In addition, the funding provided a rare research organization to conduct ongoing studies to aid the brain injured population and added to the number of neurological scientists to join the faculty at Weill Cornell Medical College in New York City.

Almost eight years have passed since that awful day and he is back to being a fun-loving dad to Noah and Andrew as he focuses on his career as well. Each day he says he is grateful to be alive.

I must admit that I have learned a lot from my son. Every doctor, but one, that treated him thought he would die. But we all saw something that we believed. He had the endurance to live and every day is dedicated to the care of his family. There is no challenge that Brad will not try to achieve and ultimate make it succeed. He shows his boys every day, how to be a better person. In fact, with trepidation, I watched him relearn how to drive with the help of Burke's personnel. It was joy to see him take himself back and forth from physical therapy to work. We would not have endured this challenge nearly as well without the support of our community. Everyone was so impressive and dedicated as well as instrumental in taking care of our family. People have their own hardships but some communities band together to help each other.

Brad was given a new perspective in his life and he saw how he could attain personal growth he was inspired and motivated. It was a collaborative effort to get him to a place of strength and endurance. People also say, "things happen for a reason." In Brad's case I could not bear to hear that phrase. What happens in your life is not luck. It is persistent and endurance to achieve your goals and Jess researched constantly to make this happen for Brad. You gain wisdom as you move forward, and you are amazed at how the body heals when the mind is in the right place. Jess looked for everything available to help him. You look for a mind and body connection. She sought out how the mind body connection affects your mental health. This is where Jess continued to seek out help. She extended herself in every way possible to secure he healed. You grasp for all that is offered to you. You spend endless hours seeking out every possible way to rehab.

When your family is at stake you stop at nothing. Nobody gets in your way. Their children learned valuable lessons that will be with them forever.

It became their life too. At their tender young ages they learned how you bond together and seek out help. It is a lesson that is critical and stays with them. Brad was given a new perspective in his life and he saw how he could attain personal growth. As a result, he was inspired and motivated. It was a collaborative effort to get him to a place of strength and endurance. What happens in your life is not luck. It is persistent and endurance to achieve your goals and Jess researched constantly to make this happen for Brad. You gain wisdom as you forge ahead, and you are amazed at how the body heals when the mind is in the right place.

CHAPTER THIRTY-FIVE

MARSHA: IN MAY of 2020, I had a brain bleed of my own and that fact alone was surreal to me. I was outdoors with Bobby by a lake near where we live, and I felt suddenly exhausted like I had a top spinning in my head when I, without thought, ran to the edge of a lake where I passed out. To this day, I have no memory of the event.

Fortunately, I live in a condominium community with an exceptional security and Emergency Medical Service that, along with Bobby, took me by ambulance to Northern Westchester Hospital in Mount Kisco. There I was scanned and surgically repaired by a staff neurosurgeon to stop the bleed. It was a lot less of an issue than Brad went through, yet I wonder how it occurred at all.

In July of that year, I went to NYU Langone for my second surgery performed by Dr. Riina. So far, I am recovering well but I was told it would take six months to a year or more heal.

Like my son, I sometimes have deep feelings of sadness, frustration, and loss, which are common traits after a brain injury. There is also a loss of energy and a lack of motivation. Self-esteem is a person's assessment of self-worth and is often adversely affected by the issue. So I was told to expect a change in behavior despite the good wishes and support that often comes from professionals and friends—all who have been there for me.

Brad always focuses on positives and expresses his feeling to whom he speaks. He directs those who he now councils to re-direct their primary feelings. When he is able to accomplish that with others, every success is huge to him as well as us.

I have learned all of this from him.

He also encourages me among others to be as independent as possible, but challenges sometimes interfere with this effort. More than anything, he wanted his independence back in every way and so do I. He has answered so many questions of those who need support to fully heal and he works hard to advise them how to enhance their lives. To this day, it surprises me that I am successfully counseled by my own son!

The way you heal, he says is with repetitive movements and professionally structured exercise. He learned that it was critical to enhance the body's endurance to recover. The whole body, in fact, has to readjust to new movements while awake and sleeping patterns which are often widely different than before the injury. Those who are not getting a full night's sleep must nap at periods in the day to enhance their brains. Listening to what your body signals is critical.

I, too, am following this series of exercises and brain reformation with a neurophysiologist and feel far better with this plan.

As time went on, Brad and I both learned that the complexity of tasks that have increased both our powers of healing, and as a result, he, particularly, developed more patience especially about spasticity.

This motor movement can range from mild to severe and that is when the patience of the person must be forthright and ongoing by ramping up the task that will allow this problem to go from severe to mild or eventually disappear.

I am in awe of son's recovery and grateful for my own. He truly became a fighter with the help of my husband Bobby, Jessica, Noah, and Andrew and of course, Dave and Vanessa. The possibilities of his recovery and mine are still endless.

He has achieved far beyond what anyone thought was possible. With the help of robotics and the exoskeleton, Brad's recovery grew by leaps and bounds not remotely expected by the doctors, therapists, and the family members.

In 2015, Brad went back to work full time. His motivation sent him on an upward track, and he continues to enjoy physical therapy with Andre and friends.

I think his sons are the proudest of him of all. "First he walked with a one-point cane and now he's on his own." Said Noah. "And my father is driving after my grandpa gave him the motivation and the keys to relearn the technique."

"Do you go driving with Daddy when he takes the car," I asked Andrew who looked upon the concept with skepticism. He simply answered, "I sit in the back seat."

Tim Hanlon, the Human Resources for GE helped support Brad with diction software and onsite support, but he was the guy who made all of the systems work. but all the Bermans found our greatest joy in paying it forward when the fundraising helped so many others.

Now I know how to play, relax, and unwind. I make lists of what nurtures me and let my inner spirit be my guide.

I also do not expect too much of myself at present because sometimes it is hard to communicate at times of crisis. During the worst of Brad's struggle, I found a way to inhale and exhale to loosen my grip on terror. Even when recovery begins, the patient, as well as the family, may become overwhelmed and all should seek help to balance their feelings.

Brain injury may make the patient feel inferior because they have lost control. Over time, balance can help everyone involved to learn relaxation techniques, remember how to intensify their sense of humor, and attempt to work at the complexity of tasks that may not have been present when the incident occurred.

That is why support groups are necessary to help family members through their traumatic experience. In this environment you are able to avoid labeling, categorizing the lack of communication skills for the injured person as well as their loved ones.

Positivity, I learned throughout our ordeal—both his and ours—is essential because every success is huge in the scheme of things. At this point in life, Brad wants to run a 5K with his sons. He also wants to play tennis again. And he wants to show everyone what a capable attorney he has become again.

At one point in his recovery, his short-term memory was so bad that he could not recall what happened 10 minutes before. But now he is just a healthy young man with a slight limp and a weak arm. As he explains, he might be the world's luckiest unlucky person.

After a brain injury there is always a loss of energy and a lack of motivation. Self-esteem is a person's assessment of self-worth and is often adversely affected by the issue. A change in behavior often comes from the support of others—professionals and friends. Brad always focuses on positives and expresses his feeling to whom he speaks. He steers those who he now counsels to re-direct their primary feelings. This is, to set the harsh realities aside and move forward. When he is able to accomplish that with others, every success is huge to him as well as us. I have learned all of this from him and expect to learn even more. Brad also encourages others to be as independent as possible, but challenges sometimes interfere with this effort. More than anything, he wanted his independence back in every way.

One of the problems that those with brain injuries endure is labeling or categorizing a communication skill, such as speech, that may be temporarily or permanently slurred or even lost.

He has answered so many questions of those who need support to fully heal and he continues to work hard to advise them how to enhance their lives with diversified means.

The way you heal, he says is with repetitive movements and professionally structured exercise. He learned that it was critical to enhance the body's endurance to recover. The whole body, in fact, has to readjust to new movements while awake and sleeping patterns which are often widely different than before the injury. He is still adjusting as he has been told will be a lifelong project.

CHAPTER THIRTY-SIX

MARSHA: AS TIME went by, Brad learned that the complexity of tasks increased his healing power and as a result, he developed more learning capacity as well as patience.

This motor movement can range from mild to severe and that is when the patience of the person must be forthright and ongoing by ramping up the task that will allow a specific problem to go from severe to mild or ultimately disappear.

Now I know how to play, relax, and unwind. I make lists of what nurtures me and let my inner spirit be my guide.

I also do not expect too much of myself at present because sometimes it is hard to communicate at times of crisis. Yet I am writing this book with the help of my editor and my sons. It is a difficult state, but during the worst of Brad's struggle, I found a way to inhale and exhale to loosen my grip on the terror. Even when recovery begins, the patient, as well as the family, may become overwhelmed and they should seek help to balance their feelings. I cannot say enough about this issue.

Brain injury may make the patient feel inferior because they have lost control. I know. It happened to me. Over time, balance can help everyone involved to learn relaxation techniques, remember how to intensify their sense of humor, and attempt to work at the complexity of tasks that may not have been present when the incident occurred.

That is why support from every segment of our personal universe is necessary to help family members through the traumatic experience. It brings to mind the lyrics of *Bridge Over Troubled Waters*. In this environment you are able to avoid labeling, categorizing the lack of communication skills for the injured person as well as their loved ones. Positivity, I learned throughout our ordeal is essential because every success is huge in the scheme of things.

Having a vision is the most powerful tool. I always perceived my sons as healthy children who grew to powerfully capable men. Happy and healthy was all I expected as Bobby and I believed that our family would bring this capability to fruition. And so we were certain that our belief would become what our children and us had worked hard to produce.

My powerful vision of this faced me hard and fast when Brad was stricken, but I knew that if we had a vision to become the best at our jobs, we can also focus or recovery and endurance.

And so it went. What I feared most in the first hundred days was about Brad's resilience to recover. Clearly, we carefully chose the best doctors to treat him and endured the stress of what he had to go through to make the difference. His recovery at all four facilities was handled with a clear vision of what the professionals would provide and what Brad could expect.

They made a terrifying challenge into triumphant success. Brad makes progress every day and he contributes this to his heroes, beginning with Natalie Dawn who if you recall, saved his life in the first ambulance. She simply would not let him die all the way through the extraordinary doctors, technicians, therapists, and support staff.

Brad also sees what others who go treatment at the four facilities go through as well. He also was amazed at his introduction to neuroscience by the professionals and he and the others relearned life as they wanted it to be, as well as he had become. Everything changed over time due to the work our heroes made us sure that focus on one step at a time would bring about success.

During the time we spent in the hospitals, we saw a lot of tragedy, and we also saw success: hundreds of patients recovered and went home to their families.

After all this time, our vision never wavered. We are even more proactive and protective overall. And the key to it all is gratitude. We stayed calm amid the chaos. As a result, I know how to fill my days and balance my needs.

Being focused is a gift of what we want to concentrate and work on. It is truly a reflection of ourselves. You must clear your mind every day, you cannot push down your feelings, it will manifest in your body if you don't expect it.

Families need to talk and set their intentions for the day and the weeks ahead as much as possible.

Do not be defensive and do not make it about yourself—Love instead!

Being in the fight and flight mode for too long wreaks havoc on our bodies.

Try to help with compassion. Seek a solution instead of complaining and finger-pointing.

We all have a choice, and it all starts with us and our willingness to take action.

Remember to disengage in the moment and just breathe!

As we learned to love ourselves and to stop looking for reasons to criticize ourselves, we found it was vital to play as well as pray; meditate and deeply breathe and routinely process your thoughts. But most of all, remember to be caring and understand the need for this behavior, especially during times of turmoil. We know turmoil. We learned kindness. We know fear; we learned courage. We do not look for praise; we live our lives to the best of our ability.

Brad tends to go way beyond, having been the one who learned these lessons best. Since his children were small when the AVM occurred, he spends a great deal of time with Noah and Andrew now in their early teens and has taught them that sometimes life deals you a hand you didn't expect, but your persevere and you get back on track. That, he says, is how you control your own destiny.

His journey taught him that if you suffer, and can change with gratitude, a sense of humor and the ability to help others with your new-found knowledge fully develops. He also learned to stay away from negative social media because we can pass this toxicity on to those we love and respect.

And that is how we all learned that his vision was our vision. As you go through life an illness or other type of tragedy may become a part of your whole life's journey. My routine includes calm mindset, healthy habits, and loving relationships. We wish for the best, knowing that things happen, and you have to be ready to resolve it with all your strength.

Things do not just happen because we wish or hope they would. My journey continues and my thirst for knowledge is never ending. Knowledge is power but having knowledge and putting it into action yields better results than wishing and hoping. Last but not least: Learn to love, enjoy, and be satisfied with the results. You will be surprised at the result.

CHAPTER THIRTY-SEVEN

HAVING A VISION is the most influential tool. I always perceived my sons as healthy children who grew to strongly capable men. Happy and healthy was all I expected as Bobby and I believed that our family would bring this capability to fruition. And so we were certain that our belief would become what our children and us had worked hard to produce.

My prevailing vision of this faced me hard and fast when Brad was stricken, but I knew that if we had a vision to become the best at our jobs, we can also focus or recovery and endurance.

And so it went. What I feared most in the first hundred days was about Brad's resilience to recover. Clearly, we had chosen the best doctors to treat him and endured the stress of what he had to go through to make the difference. His recovery at all four facilities was astounding. They all made a terrifying challenge into triumphant success.

Brad also sees what others who go treatment at the four facilities go through as well. He also was amazed at his introduction to neuroscience by the professionals and he and the others relearned life as they wanted it to be as well as he had become. Everything changed over time due to the work our heroes made us sure that focus on one step at a time would bring about success.

After all this time, our vision never wavered. We are even more proactive and protective of our friends and family. And the key to it all is gratitude. We stayed calm amid the chaos. As a result, I know how to fill my days and balance my needs with gratitude for being given the opportunity to live well.

We learned to love ourselves and to stop looking for reasons to criticize. It is also vital that you play as well as pray; meditate and deeply breathe and routinely process your thoughts But most of all, be caring and understand the need for this behavior, especially during times of turmoil. We know turmoil. We learned kindness. We know fear; we learned courage. We do not look for praise; we live our lives to the best of our ability.

Brad tends to go way beyond, having been the one who learned these lessons best. Since his children were small when the AVM occurred, he spends a great deal of time with Noah and Andrew now in their early teens and has taught them that sometimes life deals you a hand you didn't expect, but your persevere and you get back on track. That, he says, is how you control your own destiny.

In 2018, life moved on in a different way for Brad and Jess. It happens in many families: people change and move apart due to major circumstances beyond their control and so do their relationships. In 2019, Brad and Jess were amicably divorced. As sad as it appeared, they did and will always do what is best for their children. They are both satisfied with their choice and remain close friends. Every decision is made with their children in mind.

Their journey taught them that if you suffer, and can change with gratitude, a sense of humor and the ability to help others with your newfound knowledge. They also learned to stay away from negative social media because we can pass this toxicity on to those we love and respect.

As we look back at this most unique year, we have learned the importance of friends, family, and country. We must remember that our family is with us, and we stand firm and united. We are optimistic in our future, and faithful that the road ahead of us will be bright, successful, and blessed. We are strong, proud and we hope that we will finally be peaceful following this challenging time in our lives.

Life isn't about waiting for the storm to pass. It's about learning to dance in the rain.

End

PHOTO GALLERY

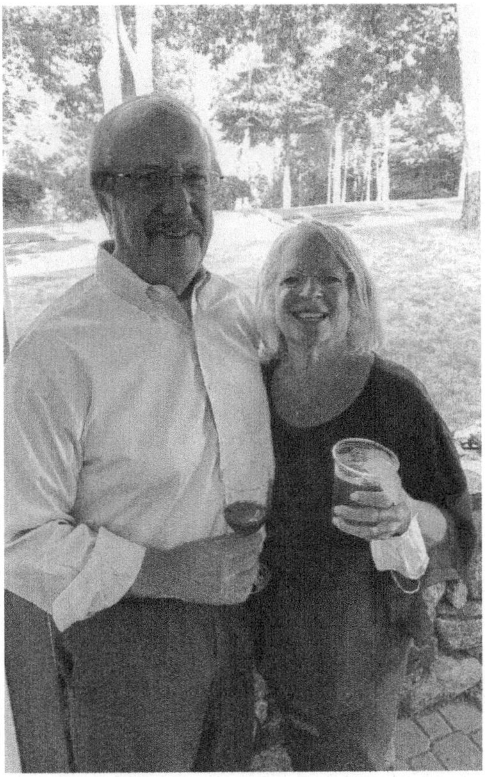

Marsha and Bob Berman-At Somers Lions Event

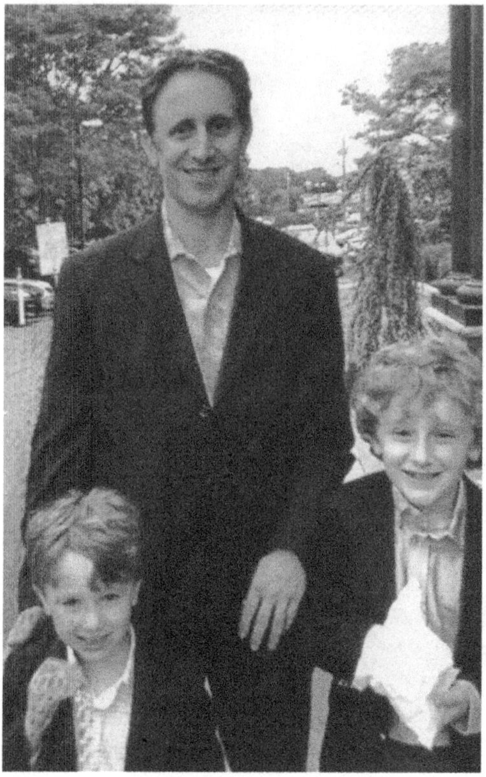

Brad Noah and Andrew

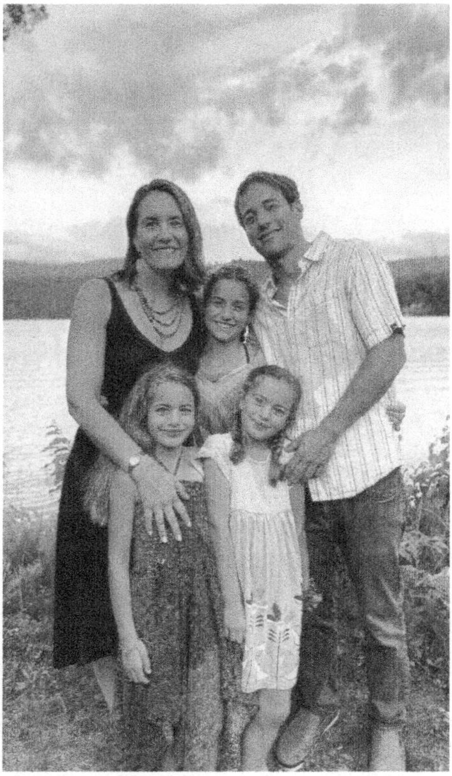

Dave, Vanessa, Alana Hazel and Sammy

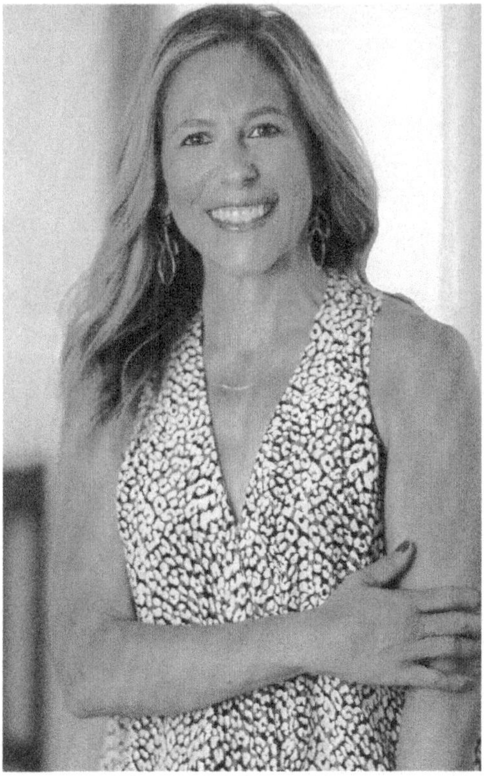

Jessica

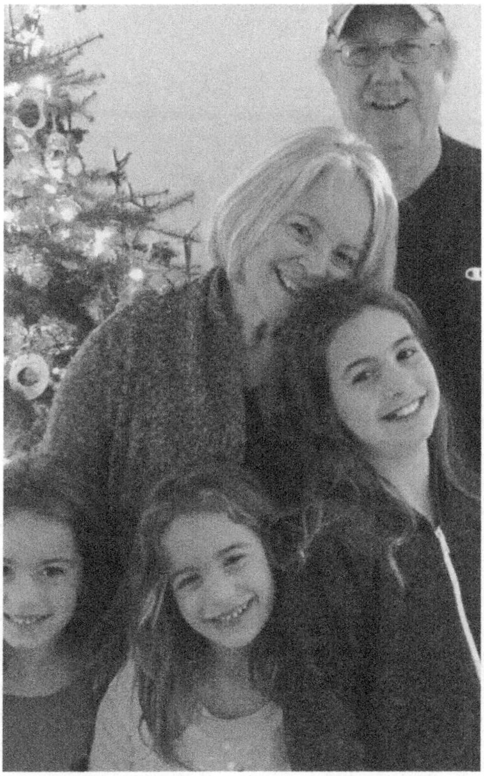

Marsha and Bob Berman and grandkids, Alana, Hazel and Sammy

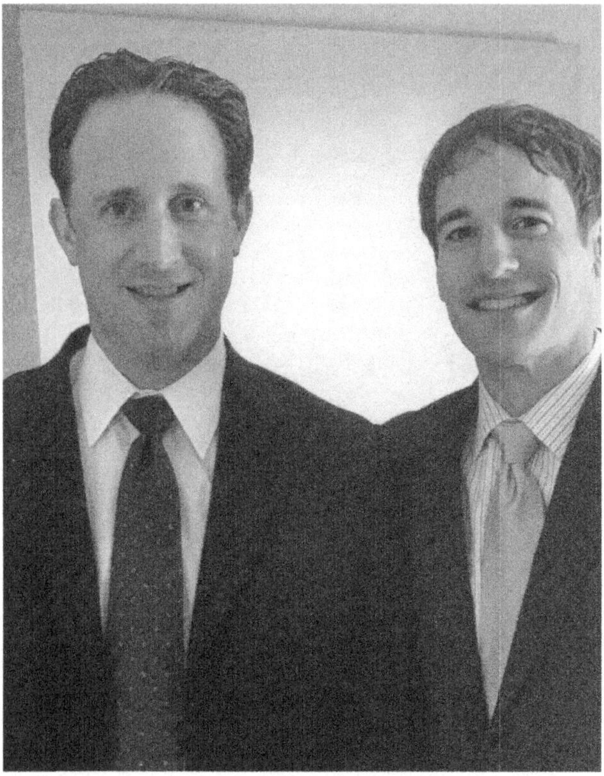

Brad and Dave

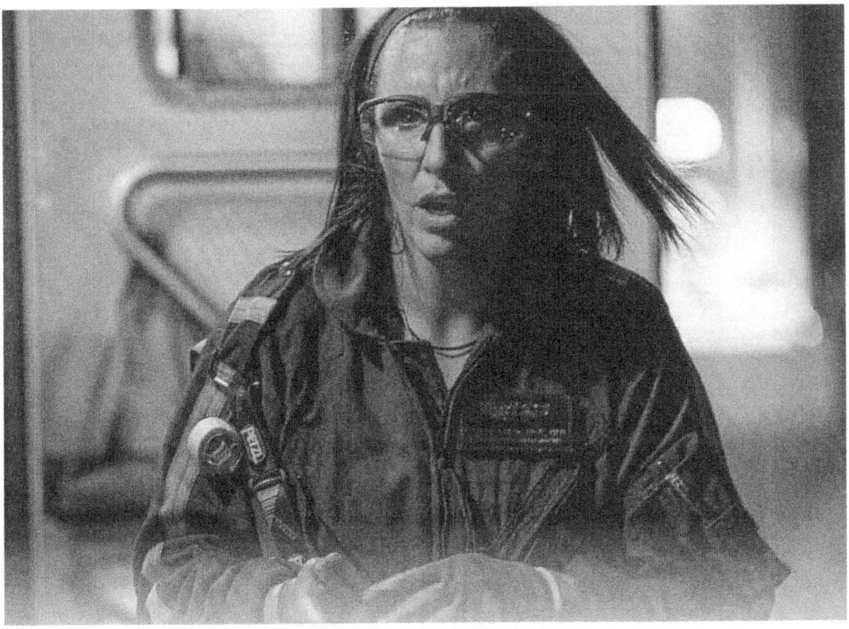

Natalie Lunde Dawn, EMS

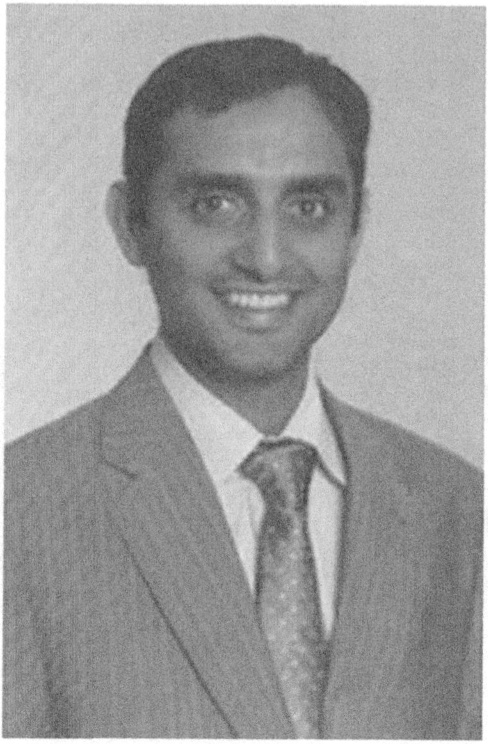

Dr. Avinash Mohan, Westchester Medical Center

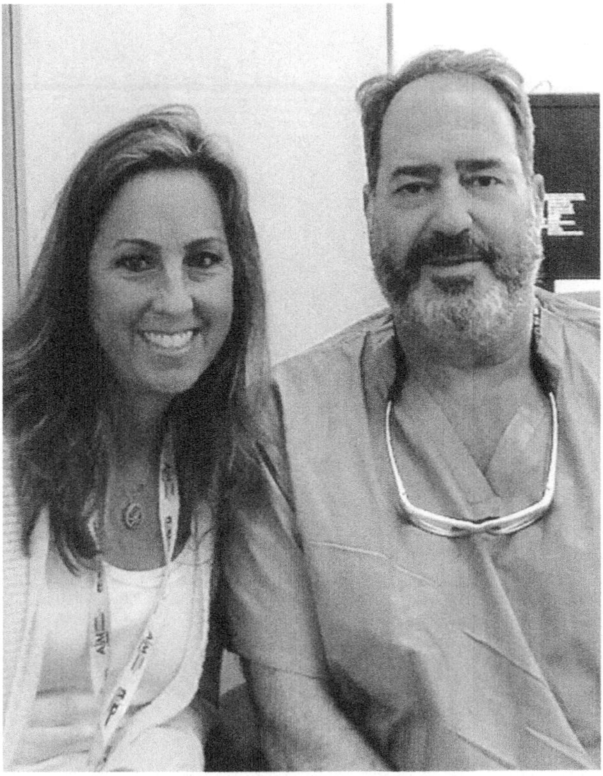

Dr. Howard Riina with Elizabeth Ponchione P.A.,
NYU Langone Medical Center

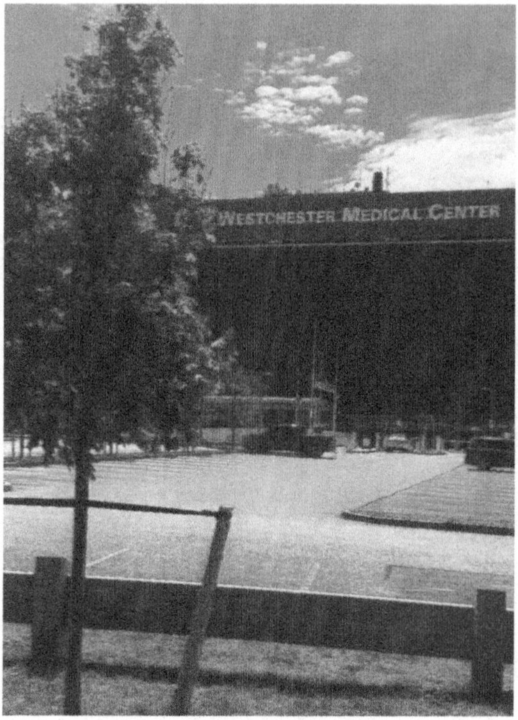

Westchester Medical Center

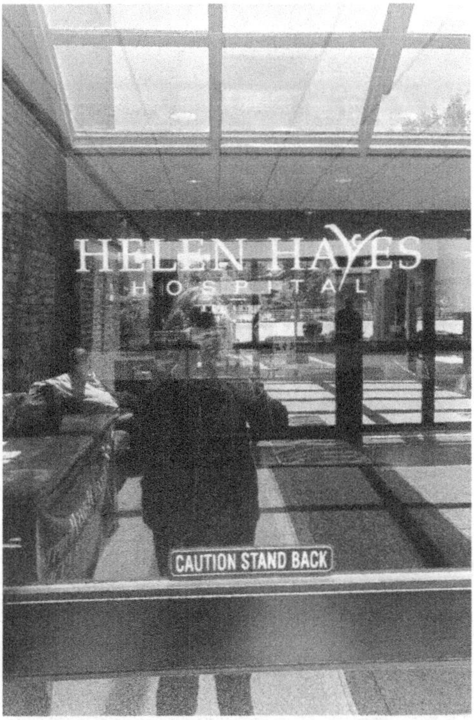

Helen Hayes Rehabilitation Center

NYU Langone Health

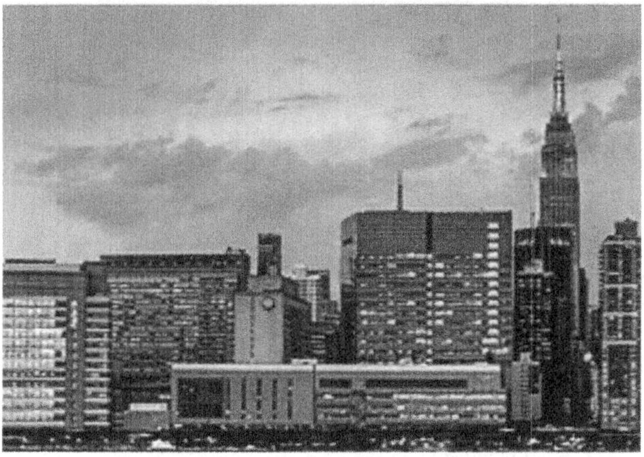

NYU Langone Medical Center

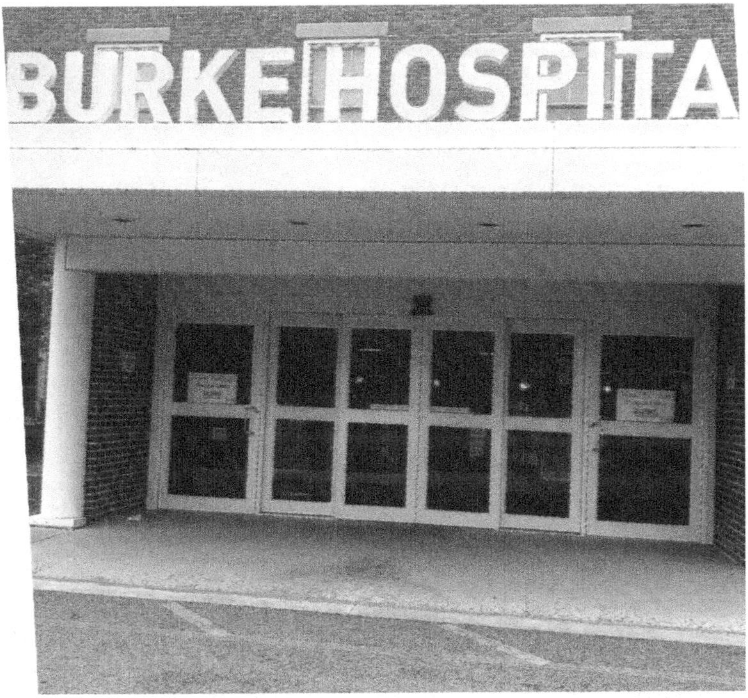

Burke Rehabilitation Center

Made in the USA
Monee, IL
06 November 2026

67974635R00080